Back-
Friendly®

A PRACTICAL GUIDE
TO PAIN RELIEF & PREVENTION

Back-Friendly®

A PRACTICAL GUIDE
TO PAIN RELIEF & PREVENTION

By JoANNE B. SCHATZ

Founder, JoAnne's Bed and Back Shops

and Linda Harris

FOREWORD BY GABE MIRKIN, M.D.

WINDY ENTERPRISES

PLEASE NOTE: The information in this book is meant to complement the advice of your physician, not to replace it. The authors stand behind the information and recommendations in this book, but because any material can be misused, the authors are not responsible for any adverse effects or consequences resulting from application of the information and recommendations. The authors expressly disclaim any liability for the use or misuse of any information contained herein. Please use this book to enhance your health, with the knowledge that you are the primary force in directing your own life and health.

For more information about JoAnne's Bed and Back Shops, or to order more copies of this book, visit our Web site at <www.backfriendly.com> or phone 1-888-SOS-BACK (1-888-767-2225).

Library of Congress Catalog Card Number 99-070810
ISBN 0-9641364-1-4

Design:	JEP Graphics
Illustrations:	Kevin Chadwick
Publisher:	Windy Enterprises
	Alexandria, VA 22314

Printed in the United States of America

*For all the people whose health and outlook
have improved after listening to my heartfelt
suggestions for relieving their pain, getting
a better night's sleep, and trying my
Back-Friendly® products.*

*And for all those whose lives I will
contribute to in the future.*

Contents

Good eating made easy ... How to use the Food Guide Pyramid ... 3 ways to exercise ... The miracle of deep breathing ... Simple ways to bring fitness to your life ... The real meaning of insomnia ... 10 tips for a good night's sleep
Summary   *38*

Back pain: a silent epidemic ... Causes of back pain ... Posture and other lifestyle elements ... Bowling ball and cup of water illustrations ... Dictionary of terms ... Your back's natural curves ... Sprains, strains, and spasms ... Disc problems
Summary   *52*

Self-treatment ... Ice and heat: contrast therapy ... 11 paths to pain relief ... Importance of moderate exercise ... Motivation for good

Foreword

JoAnne Schatz knows more than most doctors about keeping your back healthy. She attends expos and conventions regularly to learn about the latest equipment, accessories, and home and office furniture that are designed to prevent and treat back, neck, and related pain. She seeks out the expertise of physical therapists and ergonomics specialists so her clients can have the most up-to-date information. Then JoAnne matches your symptoms with the right bed, chair, back support, massager, pillow, footrest, and other "hardware" solutions.

If you already suffer from back or neck pain, JoAnne provides the best products you'll find anywhere to relieve the pain. If you have a healthy back and want to keep it that way, read this book and learn hundreds of useful tips to prevent problems with your spine.

Injuries to your spine can cause aches and pains that can be very difficult to diagnose. I regularly send my patients with back problems to JoAnne. You can benefit from her knowledge by reading *Back-Friendly* and following her recommendations.

Gabe Mirkin, M.D.
Sports medicine physician and radio talk show host

What Makes JoAnne's Special?

Hi, I'm JoAnne Schatz, president of JoAnne's Bed and Back Shops, an independently owned chain of stores specializing in products for pain relief, good sleep, and healthy living. I see myself as a problem-solver, and for more than two decades, I've dedicated my professional life to two goals: helping people prevent and overcome neck and back pain, and helping people get better, more refreshing sleep.

You might think of doctors, physical therapists, surgeons, and other health professionals as the people who provide the "software" to help you when you don't feel good. They have the training and experience to advise you how to treat that complex structure called your body. I provide the "hardware"—all the most advanced products and accessories you need to restore and maintain a healthy back, neck, and related parts of your body. My years of experience and product knowledge complement what the health professionals recommend.

In each of my stores along the Eastern Seaboard, I carry more than 1,000 products. I offer beds, mattresses, chairs, back supports, pillows, recliners, and many other Back-Help™ accessories. These include lumbar supports, car seat supports, massagers, hot and cold gel packs, and footrests. While you're in a store, you can try out anything you want, for as long as you want.

My staff are all trained by experts in ergonomics and physical therapy. Each salesperson knows the importance of good spinal alignment and good sleep, and understands what it means when you say you're in pain. When you call or visit one of the stores, you can educate yourself about any back, neck, or sleep related problems you might have. You can then discuss Back-Friendly® solutions that will ease your pain and have you feeling in tip-top shape. You can also explore ways to maintain a healthy spine and keep yourself pain free.

These solutions may be much simpler and less costly than you assume. People often walk into one of my stores expecting to make a major purchase, but after talking with the staff and learning about different options, these people walk out with a less expensive yet equally effective solution to their problem.

I constantly search for new ways to help our customers, and I always promote preventive back care as well. We assist people whose backs are healthy and who want to keep them that way. We also take care of clients with problems as complex as arthritis, fibromyalgia, and sciatica, or as common as low back pain or a stiff neck.

So you see, I really do care about you. Don't be cynical—it's true! I love to hear from customers whose pain is totally gone or who sleep much better or who have a better outlook once they've followed my advice. Some of their stories appear in this book. And after *you* come in to one of my stores, you'll experience first hand why I say: *"Your back will thank you and so do I."*

JoAnne

Acknowledgments

My beloved husband, Skip, my partner in life and in business, has patiently and enthusiastically supported me through the ups and downs of building this enterprise. We create together, we laugh together, we argue together, and we will always be together. He has my deep gratitude, my admiration, and my love.

My four wonderful children, their spouses, and my grandchildren always touch my heart. They will inherit this business someday, and I will give it to them with pride and joy.

So many others have believed in me through thick and thin. Family, friends, and shareholders have contributed money, ideas, and moral support, all of which I have needed and appreciated.

Finally, I am very grateful to all the people who work in my company, in the stores and at headquarters, for their competence, caring, and devotion to doing things the right way. Each one makes a difference in helping our customers live healthy, pain-free lives.

Thank you.

Introduction

Why You Should Read This Book

If you walk by the Health and Fitness section of a bookstore, you will see many books on back and neck care and getting a good night's sleep. Some of them have pages and pages of exercises, things to do, ways to sleep, sit, and stand—and all of this can be very confusing. How do you know which one has the best method, the most up-to-date thinking, the most practical scheme for a busy person? Do you march off to a doctor, or do you try something on your own? How do you know a new activity will be helpful and not harmful? And what if you buy an expensive piece of equipment to embark on a new exercise program, then find out the program doesn't work for you or is too complicated? Or what if you just lose interest?

Let's say you actually read one or two of these books. Now you may know something about more restful sleep or why your back hurts, but what do you do about it? How do you use your newly acquired knowledge? If you decide you need a new bed or chair, what criteria will help you choose the right one when you go shopping? What kind of product offers the best pain relief for a pulled muscle or stiff neck? What if you need some help coping with arthritis or with sciatica pain in your leg?

The book you're holding in your hands brings you the bottom line. It offers information to use in day-to-day living. Calling on my many years' experience helping people with back, neck, and sleep problems, and various pain issues, I have distilled potentially confusing solutions into an easy-to-read, simple-to-understand book. Once you read through it, applying your new knowledge will become fairly effortless. You are already motivated to get rid of pain and/or improve your health—you just need to know which direction to take. It's like reading a map; the map won't do you any good unless you see the little circle marked "You are here."

"Here" may be the crossroads of a decision about whether to buy a new mattress that will give you more restful sleep, or whether to order a chair that will help you feel more comfortable at your computer. Or "here" may be the point at which you are determined to do something to relieve the aches and pains in your back or neck that you just can't tolerate any more. Another possibility is that you are healthy and want to stay that way as your body ages. Or you may have a family member or friend who needs some help.

Information That Counts

Whatever stage you find yourself in, this book will help you determine where you are and where you want to go. Until now, you could not find a concise discussion of back, neck, sleeping, and sitting problems *along with* tried and true solutions for pain relief and greater comfort. And that's the type of information you should have at your fingertips when making your purchasing decision.

You need to know, for example, that sleeping on the cozy old pillow you used as a kid doesn't support your neck, and that you need to test several new pillows to decide which feels just right while giving you proper support. You need to know that one reason your back aches in the morning is because you toss and turn during the night, and you do *that* because the mattress and foundation of your sleep set are broken down. Again, you need to test a new set while an expert helps you figure out what works for you and what doesn't. Or you need to know that if you are short (like I am), sitting with your feet dangling instead of resting them on a supportive footrest can contribute to a backache or neck ache. You then need to make it easy to always have your feet supported by putting a footrest under your desk and carrying around a collapsible one for use in restaurants, theaters, and airplanes. I always have a portable footrest with me, and as soon as I sit down anywhere, I pull the footrest out of my handbag and set it on the floor in front of me.

So this is what my book gives you: basic, essential facts to help you make the wisest choices as you take action to nurture your spine and your overall health. It's an all-in-one book with information plus solutions for everyday living.

Determining How I Can Help You

When you come to me and say, "My lower back hurts," or "I get a stiff neck when I sit in front of my computer for a few hours," or "I have trouble sleeping through the night," here are some of the questions I might ask:

✦ When does your back usually hurt? In the morning, after driving, after work, after watching TV at home?

✦ What kind of mattress do you sleep on? How old is it? What supports the mattress?

✦ What kind of work do you do? How many hours a day are you sitting down?

✦ Do you work on a computer? How many hours a day do you spend in front of it? Do you have more than one work station?

✦ Do you read or watch TV in bed?

✦ Do you pick up heavy objects or little children?

✦ How much exercise do you get?

I ask many other questions so I can give you my very best advice on what you need to help eliminate your pain or discomfort. As you read this book, you will find much more detail about the causes and solutions for your aches and pains or your tossing and turning in bed. I encourage you to learn as much as you can, ask questions, and investigate for yourself the actions, treatments, or products that will bring you peaceful relief. You will find many real life stories; someone I write about here may have a problem just like yours.

You Are Special

I spend countless hours on customer service, making sure that people who buy from me are not only satisfied but also enthusiastic about what they're doing for themselves and how our products have helped them. I'm constantly on the phone, offering solutions and listening to my customers.

Clients have responded to my concern with wonderful feedback and gratitude. Their backaches have cleared up, their muscle pains have disappeared, or they no longer wake up grumpy in the morning because they haven't slept well. You will read stories about folks whose outlook on life literally has turned around because they no longer have that pain in their lower back or that stiff neck they left the office with every day.

I love to hear these stories and interact with people. That's really why I'm in business. Nothing brings me greater pleasure than knowing I've been able to ease someone's pain or make life a little better. Contributing to people's health gives me great satisfaction. Now I am putting what I know on paper so I can reach an even wider audience.

Dear JoAnne,

This is a letter of thanks that I have wanted to write for the past 15 years. To go back to the beginning ... I was in a car accident in early 1982 and suffered serious neck and back injuries. After long hospital stays, physical therapy, and surgeries, I was left to live with pain so severe that I could hardly function, much less sleep at night. [Getting] no sleep increased my pain, and it became a vicious cycle of agony.

After being out of commission for months, my husband offered to take me out for the afternoon. I was using a walker, and I noticed a store filled with beds. As I stood looking into the store, a nice lady by the name of JoAnne approached me. She asked if she could help me, and I said "probably not." In a voice of concern, she asked me what happened. I told her all the details.

JoAnne assisted me into her store and took me over to a bed and told me to get on the bed and make myself comfortable. It took me a while, but soon after I was so comfortable that I didn't want to move. As I lay on the bed, we chatted as though we were old friends. She told me about all the items she had that could benefit someone like myself. She had beds, chairs, bedrests, backrests, pillows—just about anything that could help someone feel better.

But you see, this was a very special store, owned by a very special person. She never sold me anything. She was not pushy or chit-chatty just to make a sale. You see, she cared about me, not the sale. After an hour or so, she asked me if I would like to take the bed home with me.

I must now brag about this bed that changed my life. It was so comfortable that I seemed to sleep forever. People would say, 'Oh, if it is that comfortable, it will be sagging in the middle before you know it.' Well, it is 15 years later, and the bed looks and feels the same as it did the day it was delivered. It is perfect!

I never forgot JoAnne. Every night, I mean every night, *I lie in bed and think about this very special lady who invited me into her store.*

—Saundra Lee Runaldue
Charlotte Hall, Md.

HOW TO USE THIS BOOK
TO YOUR BEST ADVANTAGE

✦ Check out the Table of Contents for topics that interest you most.

✦ Read chapter 1, "The Good Health Triangle," to give yourself a solid foundation for exploring ways to shape a healthier back or get a better night's sleep. I know you are eager to learn about back and sleep solutions, but don't skip this chapter. It gives extra meaning to everything else I discuss.

✦ Peruse the summaries of chapters you don't have time to read in detail right now.

✦ Note the personal stories and experiences (set in *italic* type) of the many people I have been able to help; someone's situation may be similar to yours.

✦ See the resource lists at the ends of some of the chapters and notes at the end of the book for further reading or for follow-up in an area that interests you.

✦ Use this as a workbook. Make notes in the margins and take it with you to your doctor's office or to a store when you shop for Back-Friendly products.

✦ Please try some of the solutions I recommend even if you are skeptical. They have worked for thousands of people, and they can work for you.

The Good Health Triangle

Eat Right, Exercise, Sleep Well

"We are a nation of firefighters, not fire preventers. Usually we don't fix a roof until it leaks. And usually we don't take very good care of our bodies until something goes wrong. Here's my advice: Don't operate this way anymore! Pay attention to diet, exercise, and rest, and your reward will be vibrant health for years to come."

JoAnne

HIGHLIGHTS OF THIS CHAPTER

✦ Good eating made easy

✦ How to use the Food Guide Pyramid

✦ Three ways to exercise

✦ The miracle of deep breathing

✦ Simple ways to bring fitness to your life

✦ The real meaning of insomnia

✦ Ten tips for a good night's sleep

A ll right, which is easier: correcting a problem or preventing it in the first place? In most instances, of course, prevention is the way to go. Isn't maintaining a healthy back easier than risking pain or injury that could drain your time, money, and patience to fix? The key to prevention lies in the Good Health Triangle.

The three sides of the triangle are equally important. Each lends a great deal to your overall health, but if you decide to concentrate on only one, the results will not be as dramatic or rewarding as they will be if you give yourself the gift of all three.

Eat Right

You already know a lot about the "right" way to eat, even though you may not always do it. Advertisements bombard us with messages about losing weight and eating low-fat foods. Hundreds of new fat-free or low-fat products hit the market each year. Health news and advice appear frequently on television, on radio, and in print. Many adults fight a constant battle against the creep of extra pounds, and experts warn that America's kids often spend too much time snacking on the couch in front of a TV set rather than running around outside or riding a bike.

When my husband, Skip, and I committed ourselves to a healthier, low-fat diet and regular exercise, we immediately felt better, and we also lost weight. We met Dr. Gabe Mirkin and Diana Rich, authors of *Fat Free, Flavor Full*, and we started eating the way they recommend.[1]

We concentrated on drinking eight glasses of water each day and stayed away from high-fat snacks and nibbles between meals. Some of this was pretty easy; some of it required a determined attitude. I gave up soft drinks, for example, and I really don't miss them. I now carry a water bottle with me practically everywhere I go, and I always have one on my desk at work. And if I feel like munching on something, I reach for the pretzel bag instead of the potato chips. Then when I'm out for a special occasion or when I feel like treating myself, it's okay to take a small portion of some lavish dessert or grab some french fries if I'm starved and there's nothing around but fast food.

Balance has become a motto for me, and it really works. I look to maintain my life on an even keel, to avoid doing anything to excess. The concept of balance pervades Eastern cultures. A basic principle of Oriental medicine points out that the body always seeks equilibrium and will try to compensate for anything that occurs outside the norm. So to maintain my own equilibrium, I eat the foods that nourish my body, I exercise regularly (I'm neither a marathon runner nor a "weekend athlete"), and I get the amount of sleep I need to feel good.

The Food Guide Pyramid

The U.S. Department of Agriculture (USDA) has published a practical, reasonable set of research-based guidelines to help you achieve balance in your eating. The Food Guide Pyramid helps you choose what and how much to eat from each of several food groups. Making the appropriate choices will give you the nutrients you need without excess calories, fat, sugar, or sodium. The pyramid allows you to focus on reducing total fat and also on cutting saturated fat. This lessens the chances of getting illnesses such as heart disease, diabetes, and some cancers and helps maintain a healthy weight.

The pyramid provides an outline of what to eat each day.[2] It's not intended to be a weight-loss diet; it's a life-enhancing diet that puts the brakes on high-calorie, high-fat foods. The pyramid opens possible ways to eat and invites you to exercise your imagination within fairly broad, healthy guidelines. The triangular form of the pyramid fits right in with the concept of balance: you can't balance anything without a solid base. The pyramid's base consists of bread, cereal, rice, and pasta—foods that just about everyone enjoys and already eats every day.

The pyramid specifies a range of servings within all the food groups. Your next question, then, is, What constitutes a serving? The USDA has that information, too (see "How to Use the Food Guide Pyramid" below). Notice that

Food Guide Pyramid
A Guide to Daily Food Choices

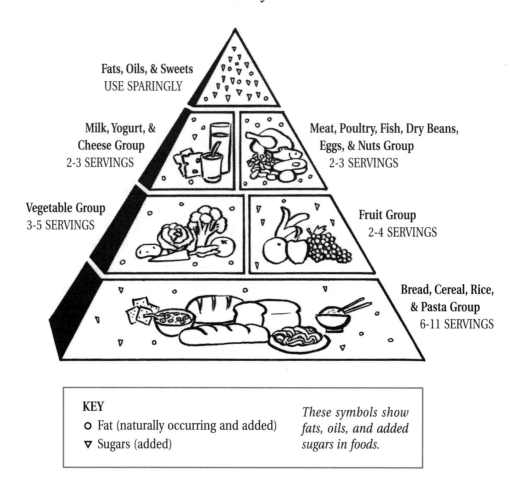

Fats, Oils, & Sweets
USE SPARINGLY

**Milk, Yogurt, &
Cheese Group**
2-3 SERVINGS

**Meat, Poultry, Fish, Dry Beans,
Eggs, & Nuts Group**
2-3 SERVINGS

Vegetable Group
3-5 SERVINGS

Fruit Group
2-4 SERVINGS

**Bread, Cereal, Rice,
& Pasta Group**
6-11 SERVINGS

KEY
o Fat (naturally occurring and added)
▽ Sugars (added)

*These symbols show
fats, oils, and added
sugars in foods.*

there is no serving size for Fats, Oils, & Sweets because the advice is to eat these "sparingly." Unless you keep an eye on these foods, "sparingly" can quickly turn into "more than enough." Here's an example: One tablespoon of just about any type of oil contains approximately 14 grams of fat. The average adult should consume about 65 grams of fat each day, so if you eat a salad with only 2 tablespoons of dressing, that uses up almost half your ideal daily fat quota! There are many ways to use oil sparingly, from low-fat or no-oil salad dressings, to cooking with just a dash of oil and adding fat-free chicken broth, water, and herbs to enhance flavor.

How to Use the Food Guide Pyramid
What Counts as One Serving?

Breads, Cereals, Rice, & Pasta
(6–11 servings per day)
1 slice bread (usually weighs
1 ounce)
$1/2$ cup cooked rice or pasta
$1/2$ cup cooked cereal
1 ounce ready-to-eat cereal

Vegetables
(3–5 servings per day)
$1/2$ cup chopped raw or cooked
vegetables
1 cup raw leafy vegetables
1 medium potato
1 medium carrot
$3/4$ cup (6 ounces) vegetable juice

Fruits
(2–4 servings per day)
1 piece fruit or melon wedge
$1/2$ grapefruit

$3/4$ cup juice
$1/2$ cup canned fruit
$1/4$ cup dried fruit

Milk, Yogurt, & Cheese
(2–3 servings per day)
1 cup milk or yogurt
$1^1/2$–2 ounces cheese

Meat, Poultry, Fish, Dry Beans,
Eggs, & Nuts
(2–3 servings per day)
$2^1/2$–3 ounces cooked lean meat,
poultry, or fish
($1/2$ cup cooked beans, 1 egg,
or 2 tablespoons peanut butter
equals 1 ounce lean meat)

Fats, Oils, & Sweets
Use sparingly, especially if you
want to lose weight

Now, that's not so difficult, is it? You probably already eat the minimum amount in each of these categories, and in some categories, you may exceed the minimum. In the United States, a typical serving of meat or poultry tips the scale at 6 to 7 ounces, not 3. Two ounces of cheese mounts up quickly when you're out for pizza or lasagna. In the grain category, that nice fresh bagel you pick up on your way to work can weigh about 6 ounces, so that's six servings right there (and 500 calories in some instances). Eating by the pyramid becomes a snap, though, when you practice it for a while. And remember, if you are trying to lose weight, fill up on fruits, vegetables, whole grains, and legumes (dried beans).

When you choose your meals based on the Food Guide Pyramid, I promise that you will have more energy and that you will just feel better about yourself and your health. A bonus of healthy eating is good elimination, or healthy bowels. And this can be very important for your back. If low back pain has already sensitized the nerves in that area, a build-up of toxins in the bowels can increase stress levels and refer pain to the back.

By the way, if you've been a "yo-yo dieter" for many years, I have a new approach to recommend. Yo-yo dieting means you lose some weight, say 5, 10, or even 15 pounds or more, by means of a diet you are really committed to and really like. But you can't keep the weight off, and you gain it back. You return to a strict diet, either the same plan or a different one, lose the weight again, then gain it back again once the strict diet ends. Some people do this

Bob G. had been overweight for most of his 60 years. Not only did he get more than his share of the flu and other illnesses, but he also constantly complained about his aching back. He hardly exercised, and he could not walk up the stairs in his home without panting.

When Bob's wife pointed out the benefits of the Food Guide Pyramid to him, the two of them chose to start eating according to its guidelines. Bob saw his doctor and began an exercise program. And with very little effort, he gradually lost his excess weight, gained more energy, and felt much better about himself. His back felt better, and the next winter, he didn't even get sick!

their entire lives! Can you imagine how frustrating this is, and how rough it is on self-esteem?

The new idea I have for you comes from the book *Intuitive Eating: A Recovery Book for the Chronic Dieter*, by two nutritionists, Evelyn Tribole and Elyse Resch.[3] Intuitive eating is what children do naturally: They eat when they're hungry and quit when they're full. They instinctively know what foods nourish their growth, so even if they don't eat a lot of vegetables, for example, they get equivalent nutrients from other foods such as fruits, nuts, and grains. *Intuitive Eating* has some wonderful information and advice on rejecting the "diet mentality," making peace with food, and challenging the "food police"—those voices in your head that tell you what you can and cannot eat. If you've had it with diets and you're feeling bad about your weight, give this a try.

Keeping Fit

The second side of the Good Health Triangle is exercise. You may already be doing it. Or you may be sick and tired of hearing how you should be doing it. Or you may want to do it but can't quite make it happen. In any case, getting enough exercise has become a vital aspect of living a healthy life. Study after study proves that exercise helps you feel better, avoid illness, and live longer. And the good news is that you can begin regular exercise at any age and reap incredible benefits. People in their eighties have started light weightlifting and moderate aerobic activity, and research studies show immediate benefits to their health.[4]

You don't have to be an Olympic athlete. Just be active enough to get your heart pumping, your pores sweating, and your muscles passing through as full a range of motion as they can without pain or injury. The U.S. Surgeon General's Report on Physical Activity and Health (1996) advises that physical inactivity poses a major health hazard, equivalent to smoking, high blood pressure, and high cholesterol. The report also concludes, as do many other new studies, that almost any exercise, even at moderate intensity, can provide major health benefits, including longer life, reduced risk of heart disease, preven-

When my neighbor wanted to start exercising, her daughter volunteered to help her, and they began to walk each morning, rain or shine, for half an hour. They worked up to 45 minutes a morning and also increased the pace. They would go until they were both breathing hard, but could still chatter. They both reported that they felt great, and my neighbor's backaches disappeared!

tion of osteoporosis, and help for arthritis sufferers.

The report's recommendations call for at least 30 minutes of moderate activity each day, and these 30 minutes don't even have to be all at once! You could do 10 minutes of housekeeping chores, walk briskly for 10 minutes, and shoot a few baskets with your kid—and you'd be set, at least to meet the minimum standard. Don't expect to lose weight by engaging only in moderate activities, however. A weight-loss program requires a higher level of exercise and attention to your calorie intake.

Please recognize that while housework or a brisk walk with the dog counts as exercise, so do 45 minutes on the treadmill or a 5-mile run. If you are in shape and are accustomed to that run or that treadmill walk, your body will benefit all the more from these more vigorous workouts. I'm *not* advising you to cut back on exercise if you are already in the habit of exercising more than 30 minutes. But if you are just beginning an exercise program, or if you are older and more sedentary, then yoga, housework, dogwalking, or gardening can give you an all-over glow from feeling proud and healthy.

Another Trio: Three Ways to Exercise

I always say, "If you're going to do something, do it right." That's the way I treat my customers, my friends, my family, and myself. So when you start or revamp your exercise program, do it right. Include the following three essential components of exercise:

+ Aerobics
+ Muscle toning and strength training
+ Stretching

Doing only one or two of these without the others won't really give you the results you want. As my doctor once said, "What good is it to be able to do 45 minutes of aerobics if the rest of your muscles aren't strong enough to lift a bag of groceries without putting a strain on your heart?" He was exaggerating, of course, but the point is that each of the components supports the other two.

Aerobics

The heart is a muscle, so it needs to be flexed and exercised just like the rest of your muscles. Some form of aerobic exercise for at least 20 minutes three times a week will keep your heart muscle in good shape. A little more, such as 30 minutes 4 to 5 days a week, would be even better; significantly less just won't give you the health benefits you want. As you know, aerobics can mean a class at the gym, a brisk walk, or a workout on a piece of equipment such as a treadmill or a cross-country skiing machine. The object is to get your "target" heart rate to within about 70–75 percent of your maximum heart rate and keep it there for at least 20 minutes. (Depending on your own health, capabilities, and goals, your target could be anywhere from 60-85 percent of your maximum heart rate.)

Here's the way to calculate your target heart rate. Subtract your age from 220. This is your maximum heart rate, the rate you don't want to exceed. Multiply this number by .75, and you will have your ideal exercise rate, your 75 percent "target" while you exercise. If you multiply by .60 or .70, then you will have the 60 percent or 70 percent rate.

For example, if you are 55 years old, here's how you would calculate the 75 percent rate:

$$
\begin{array}{r}
220 \\
-\underline{55} \\
165 \\
\times\underline{.75} \\
124 \\
\end{array}
$$

165 *(maximum heart rate)*

124 *(target heart rate)*

There's another way to estimate your exercise intensity with the Rate of Perceived Exertion (RPE) scale. Your fitness center or gym probably has a wall chart showing a scale from 0 (no perceived exertion) to 10 (very, very heavy exertion). Most people can exercise comfortably and effectively in the 3 to 5 range of perceived exertion. The RPE provides a technique for exercisers to monitor their heart rates without having to stop and count the pulse. If you are just beginning an exercise program, however, you may want to keep closer tabs on your heart rate with a monitor or a pulse count.

Muscle Toning and Strength Training

Putting your body through a toning and training routine doesn't mean you will automatically look like those pumped-up bodybuilders you see on TV. But it does mean you will improve your body's muscle-to-fat ratio by building and preserving muscle mass, which in turn increases calorie-burning efficiency and reduces body fat. When you first start a strength-training program, you may not lose weight—you may even gain. But that is because your muscle fibers themselves are expanding. When combined with cardiovascular exercise and proper eating, the fat starts to disappear and your weight goes into your muscles.

It is important to maintain the proper balance among your various muscle groups. For example, your back muscles need to be about 20 to 30 percent stronger than your abdominal muscles to give your body the right posture and prevent back pain. If you use exercise machines that have different resistance settings, you can establish the appropriate ratios for your different muscle groups. If your program uses flexible rubber bands, tubing, or free weights, you can still figure out the proper resistance for each muscle group.

A key point to remember is that you need to make your muscles strong either on machines that offer resistance or through weight-bearing exercise, or by using the resistance that gravity offers. So you might want to combine aerobics and weight bearing by walking, running, line dancing, playing tennis, or doing whatever turns you on. Weight-bearing exercise is especially important for women who need to maintain bone mass as one way to prevent osteoporosis.

Stretching

In the classic bestseller *Stretching,*[5] author Bob Anderson says that stretching provides the link between the sedentary life and the active life. It keeps the muscles supple, helps prevent injuries when you exercise, develops body awareness, and promotes circulation. Moreover, Anderson says:

"Stretching is not stressful. It is peaceful, relaxing, and non-competitive. It is completely adjustable to the individual. You do not have to conform to any unyielding discipline; stretching gives you the freedom to be yourself and enjoy being yourself." (p. 9)

What more could you want? Stretching reduces muscle tension and makes you feel more relaxed. Strenuous exercise or single-discipline exercise can lead to tightness and inflexibility because you may use only one muscle group over and over. For overall fitness, you must stretch all the major muscle groups. Don't worry—it doesn't take very long. You could identify 8–10 stretches you like, stretches that make you feel good. Hold each of them for a minimum of 10–30 seconds, and you'll be finished in less than 10 minutes. (Chapter 3 includes more stretching tips.)

Fitness experts now recommend that you warm up your muscles a bit even before you stretch, because stretching a cold, tight muscle could cause it to tear. So ideally, you would do a brief (5-10 minute), low-impact aerobic warm-up, then stretch, then do your 20-minute (or more) aerobic exercise, then stretch again to loosen the muscles and help them recover.

Here are some do's and don'ts for stretching:

+ Don't bounce.
+ Do hold the stretch for 10–30 seconds.
+ Don't stretch if it is truly painful.
+ Probably the most important "do" is breathe!

Breathe slowly, fully, and deeply, inhaling and exhaling as you change patterns of movement. Inhaling brings more oxygen to your muscles and entire bloodstream; exhaling releases carbon dioxide and other toxins. The lungs themselves have no muscles, so in order to keep them strong and capable of taking in enough oxygen, the muscles in the abdomen are used to push the lungs up and out. "Abdominal breathing" is a cornerstone of yoga and other exercise and relaxation disciplines. When you breathe this way, you can watch your abdomen rise as you inhale and fall as you exhale. It may look and feel like the opposite of what you've been doing all along, but trust me, it's the healthiest way to go.

My sister-in-law seems to use every spare moment to stretch some part of her body. She stretches while she's talking on the phone, or watching television, or even waiting in line (a discreet circling of her ankle, perhaps). Her reward is a flexible body that contributes to her overall health.

Deep, abdominal breathing is really an exercise all by itself. It brings incalculable benefits to your entire body, leads to stress reduction and relaxation, and can give you a sense of peace and appreciation for life that you may not have experienced before.

Some Easy Ways to Incorporate Fitness into Your Life

- ✦ Walk each day with someone in your family or with a neighbor.
- ✦ Walk up stairs instead of taking the elevator or escalator.
- ✦ Toss a ball around with a kid.
- ✦ Vacuum your entire house.
- ✦ Walk 20 minutes to a bagel shop on your lunch hour, buy a bagel with a low-fat spread, and walk back to work.
- ✦ Sit on the floor and stretch as you watch TV.
- ✦ Help a friend clean out the attic.
- ✦ Ride a bike for an hour or two.
- ✦ Take the tennis lessons you've always wanted.
- ✦ Park at the opposite end of the mall from where you really want to shop.
- ✦ Invent your own activities!

Last but Not Least: Sleep Well

The third side of the Good Health Triangle is allowing yourself a good night's sleep. Getting enough good, quality sleep is so important I will devote more space to it later in this book (see chapter 5). I'm sure you already know how important it is for you. You've probably had times when you couldn't fall asleep, when you've tossed and turned during the night, or when you've awakened in the morning feeling groggy and tired. A 1995 Gallup Poll reports that nearly half of all Americans say they've had trouble sleeping at one time or another. Four out of 10 insomniacs report medicating themselves to get to sleep, most often with alcohol, nonprescription sleep aids, and aspirin.[6] (In fact, you'll read below that alcohol actually *detracts* from good sleep.)

Insomnia means not getting enough sleep to meet the needs of your body or to allow you to feel refreshed and energetic upon awakening. The consequences of insomnia can range from mild daytime drowsiness to serious injuries or even death in an accident. Some accidents occur when people who haven't had enough sleep lose their concentration while driving or operating machinery. Research shows that a night of disturbed sleep can significantly affect energy level, mood, and mental dexterity.

So how do you ensure that you get enough sleep to keep you healthy and happy? The Better Sleep Council offers 10 tips for a good night's sleep.[7] This is common-sense information that everyone knows but probably ignores from time to time.

10 Tips for a Good Night's Sleep

1. *Keep regular hours.* Try to go to sleep and get up at about the same times each day, even on weekends. This schedule regulates your biological clock and gives your body a rhythm. If you stay up really late on Saturday night and sleep in on Sunday, you probably won't be able to go to sleep at your normal time on Sunday night, and that will throw off your schedule for a day or two.

2. *Develop a sleep ritual.* When you do the same things each night before you go to bed, your body knows what's next: sleep. You may want to take a warm bath, read something that is not too stimulating, do some gentle stretches or breathing exercises, or have a quiet talk with your mate. Whatever you do that works for you is fine—just do it regularly.

3. *Sleep on a good bed.* People tend to get used to their beds, and they may not realize when the bed starts losing its support and resiliency. See chapter 6 for information on how to determine whether you need a new bed and how to buy a new mattress.

4. *Exercise regularly.* Where have you heard this before? As you know, exercise not only stimulates your body, but also relaxes it from the tensions that build up during the day. If you exercise too close to bedtime, you won't feel like going to sleep. Some people like to exercise first thing in the morning; for others, the ideal time to work out is in the late afternoon or early evening.

5. *Cut down on stimulants.* North Americans drink millions of cups of coffee a day, to say nothing of the caffeine we consume in sodas, teas, and chocolate. Some people claim they can fall right asleep despite a late evening cup of coffee, but for most, caffeine is an eye opener rather than a relaxant. Other stimulants, including some drugs or diet pills, may interfere with sleep.

   Even watching late night television can be too stimulating! Dr. Andrew Weil, a respected practitioner of natural and preventive medicine, recommends a "news fast" as part of a self-healing program that includes getting good, quality sleep.[8] He suggests refraining from reading, watching, or listening to any news for a day and then checking in with your feelings. You can increase the number of days for your news fast, too. When I'm on vacation, I hardly hear any news at all, and I don't seem to suffer from that one bit.

6. *Don't smoke.* Nicotine is an even stronger stimulant than caffeine. Research shows that heavy smokers take longer to fall asleep, wake up more often, and spend less time in deep sleep. When smokers quit, their sleep

improves dramatically. So, to all the other health benefits of not smoking, add the benefit of better sleep.

7. ***Drink alcohol in moderation.*** Many people think that a glass of wine or a drink before bedtime relaxes them, but it actually disturbs normal sleep patterns. Alcohol can make it harder for you to fall asleep or stay asleep; it disturbs sleep activity in the brain. Remember the Oriental concept of letting your body find its balance, and use alcohol appropriately.

8. ***Set aside time to worry or plan early in the evening.*** If you're one of those people who lie in bed thinking about what happened today or what you need to do tomorrow, try to plan another time to do this. When you go to bed, tell your mind it's time to rest. Do some relaxation exercises or deep breathing, and let your mind wander to pleasant thoughts or images.

9. ***Create a restful sleep environment.*** Sleep in a cool, quiet, dark room on a comfortable, supportive mattress and foundation.

10. ***Make sleep a priority.*** Say yes to sleep even when you are tempted to stay up late. You will thank yourself in the morning.

Heather B., 52 years old, began having problems staying asleep at night. She had always been a good sleeper, but as she experienced menopause, she developed a common problem of women her age: sleep disturbances. She started waking up in the middle of the night with her mind racing, and she couldn't get back to sleep. After talking with her doctor and her friends, she decided to take action to get her sleep back on track.

Heather enrolled in an early evening yoga class, which she found very relaxing. She remained relaxed and quiet throughout the evening, and before going to bed, she drank some chamomile tea and did a few deep breathing exercises. During the day, Heather started writing her concerns and things to do on lists that she kept handy, so by the end of the day, she knew she could stop worrying about those things. She established a bedtime routine and soon began to sleep through the night again.

SUMMARY

I always get inspired when I read or talk about the benefits of eating right, exercising regularly, and sleeping well. It's not that I'm perfect nor do I always pay attention to all three of these critical factors for good health and long life. But I strive to keep them a big part of my life, because I *know* I'll feel better when I do.

Here's what you need to remember for good health:

◆ Base your diet on healthy grains, vegetables, and fruits, with moderate portions of dairy and other protein foods (meat, poultry, fish, eggs, nuts, beans) each day. Use fats, oils, and sweets very sparingly.

◆ Get at least 30 minutes of moderate exercise each day; higher intensity is even better if you are accustomed to it.

◆ Keep a regular sleep schedule, listening to your body as it tells you how much sleep you need to feel rested and refreshed.

Now that you are familiar with the Good Health Triangle and its role in the prevention of illness, let's look at the nature of back problems and some very practical solutions.

CHAPTER 2

Back and Neck Pain 101
Why You Hurt

"Eight out of 10 people—that's 80 percent of the population—will experience some form of back pain in their lifetime. My goal is to help prevent and lessen that pain."

JoAnne

HIGHLIGHTS OF THIS CHAPTER

✦ Back pain: a silent epidemic

✦ Causes of back pain

✦ Posture and other lifestyle elements

✦ Bowling ball and cup of water illustrations

✦ Dictionary of terms

✦ Your back's natural curves

✦ Sprains, strains, and spasms

✦ Disc problems

Back pain can occur in many ways—from waking up a little stiff to twisting a bit too much when you try to return a tennis ball, from lifting a carton that's too heavy to pulling open a door that doesn't want to budge.

Back pain can result from something major, such as an auto accident or pregnancy, or from something seemingly minor, such as bending down to pick up a pencil from the floor. Or you may not even know what caused your pain; for some people, it seems to happen without cause or explanation.

When I talk about back pain, I'm also including your neck. Neck pain usually doesn't happen in an instant (although it may). Rather, it is typically the result of something more long term, such as always cradling the phone between your ear and your neck so you can talk "hands free," or sleeping without proper support from your pillow and mattress. Stress often appears as a big culprit, because it can pile up as muscular pain, which can then translate into a tension headache or shoulder pain.

So pain can occur in any part of your spine, and often the pain in an arm or leg has its source in the spine. Each year, back pain strikes another 7 to 8 million people, leaving about 2 million totally disabled. A 1995 study shows that during any given month, more than one-third of all adults report they have back pain.[1] If that many people griped about some other malady, such as acne or the flu, it would be labeled an epidemic, and lots of money would be spent investigating and eradicating it.

Though back pain is a more silent "epidemic," it is the second leading cause of worker absenteeism in the United States, and it is responsible for a lot of complaints around the water cooler at work or the kitchen table at home! And if *you* have ever been the victim of such pain, you know it is one of the most aggravating things that can happen to you. You don't feel sick, but you just can't move very easily.

Lifestyle: A Big Chunk of the Bottom Line

Marjorie Werrell, president of Ergoworks Consulting in Gaithersburg, Md., says that 60 percent of back problems stem from bad habits such as

- Years of poor posture
- Improper body mechanics
- Stressful living and working conditions
- Poor nutrition
- Lack of flexibility
- Poor fitness

All these are 100 percent under your control; so instead of complaining, do something about it! That's what much of this book is about.

The Aging Spine

When you are young, you can recover fairly quickly from minor backaches and pains or muscle spasms. But as you age, the spine's shock-absorbing discs begin to dehydrate and lose flexibility, thus increasing the susceptibility to injury and pain. In older people, recovery takes longer each time they strain or injure the back. Add to this the fact that many people exercise less and gain some weight as they age—which puts additional strain on the back—and you have the potential for major ongoing pain.

The good news is that you can successfully treat almost all back problems yourself with some knowledge and the proper tools. The treatment may be as simple as finding the right chair or mattress, or learning how to protect your back when you bend down or pick things up. You may need to rearrange your work station or put a lumbar support in your car. Products designed to

I get such a thrill out of seeing people smile with relief when I can help them ease their pain. A truck driver looking for something that would alleviate his constant low back ache came into one of my stores. He tested several lumbar support cushions in his vehicle and bought the one that felt just right. Several days later, he stopped by, grinning from ear to ear, to tell me that he'd never been so comfortable in his truck since he started using the backrest.

help you maintain good posture while sitting or lying down can provide almost immediate relief from backaches and neck aches. Combine these products with some well-designed exercises, lose those extra 12 pounds you've been carrying around, or learn some proven relaxation techniques, and your body could feel like new in no time. Of course, if a problem persists, you need to see a doctor. But in general, my first recommendation to you is to take care of yourself! Learn how to prevent back and neck pain, and if you do have a problem, learn how to relieve it. You will be amazed at how the smallest changes can have a big impact on how you feel.

Why Does Your Back Ache?

Back pain often means you've strained some muscles and damaged the tissue. Everyday activities can be the culprits, or you may have special circumstances such as these:

+ Auto accidents or injuries at work or at play often top the list.
+ Lack of exercise, bad posture, and poor body position (body mechanics) when lifting can also precipitate a bout of pain.
+ Overeating, chronic coughing, or your heredity may play a role.
+ Tension often translates into pain in the mid-region of your back.
+ Pregnancy often causes back pain because the baby's extra weight puts a strain on the mother's lower back.
+ "Weekend athletes" who don't exercise during the work week but who exert themselves on their days off can end up in bad shape by Monday morning.
+ The longest, largest nerve in your body, the sciatic nerve, can be inflamed (sciatica) and send sharp pains into the buttocks, legs, or feet.

Some people visit a medical professional—an orthopedist, chiropractor, neurologist, or family doctor—before they come to me; others come to me first when they are seeking relief. I ask about their activities and lifestyle before I recommend simple remedies for their pain. Here are just a few of the questions I typically ask:

- ✦ Do your mattress and pillow give good support as you sleep? (Your spine should be in a straight line, so your pillow should fill in the empty space at your neck.)

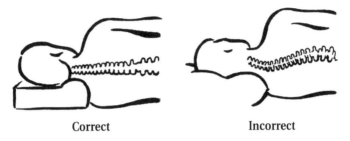

Correct   Incorrect

- ✦ Do you clench your jaw or grind your teeth as you work or sleep? (These can lead to neck pain and jaw problems known as TMJ.)
- ✦ What do you do for exercise and relaxation?
- ✦ Do you work in front of a computer? Are your feet on the floor? Is your head in line with your shoulders, as if a rope hanging straight down from the sky to the top of your head could pull you right up? (People often work in a "C" position, with their neck forward and back curved.)

Imagine Your Head as a Bowling Ball

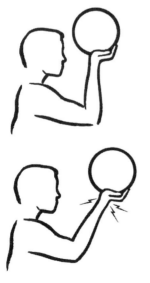

If you have neck pain, maybe this example will help you understand why.[2] Your head weighs about 14 pounds, and so do many bowling balls. Pretend you have a bowling ball in your hand, with your wrist bent back and your arm sticking up in the air from your elbow resting on a table. When you move your hand forward, consider the enormous strain this movement puts on your wrist and arm! A similar strain can go into your neck if you are sitting incorrectly at your computer, for example, or standing in poor posture.

Just Living Takes Its Toll

Perhaps the greatest contributor to back and neck pain is simple wear and tear, the pounding your back takes all day, every day, from standing, walking, or driving a car. Even just sitting still can distress your back if you don't sit in a supportive position because the weight of your torso, arms, shoulders, and head adds to the stress on your lower back. Dr. Mark Smith, a chiropractor practicing in Vienna, Va., says, "The absolute worst thing you can do is to put a static load on your back for a long period of time." "Static" means not moving from your position, whether it is sitting or standing. Whether we sit or stand, gravity exerts a tremendous force, literally pulling our vertebrae together toward the center of the earth. The secret to relieving and preventing pain lies in learning how to minimize all this strain.

Have you ever wondered why bars in restaurants or saloons have a brass rail around them, a few inches off the floor? In the "old days," cowboys and other customers used this rail to prop up one foot, so they could stand for hours without hurting their backs! Propping up one foot as you stand takes pressure off the spine and encourages proper curvature of the upper and lower back.

My "Cup of Water" Lesson

Maybe you're one of those people who get a little stabbing pain in your back and you say, "It'll go away—I'll just ignore it." And maybe it does go away. But it might return, even in another area of your back or neck, or it might get worse. Each little incident accumulates in what I call your "cup of troubles." Think of a leaky faucet that keeps dripping into a cup that can hold only a finite amount of water. At some point, the water starts overflowing. By the same token, you can fill your back to a certain extent with little aches and pains and not feel any ill effects or have any major problems. Eventually, however, the cup will overflow. You then get a major pain and can't straighten up, and all of a sudden you're in the hospital, contemplating back surgery.

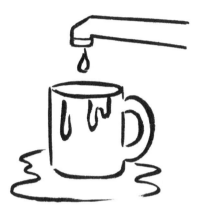

Of course not everyone's cup overflows, but this analogy does demonstrate the danger of not attending to the proper care of your back. You could wake up in the morning and have so much back pain that you can't get out of bed. You might wonder, "What did I do to have this happen?" And you can't think of anything you did last night or yesterday that might have caused such agony. But it might just be the net result of loading all those problems into your cup until they finally spill over the top in one big "ouch." Or maybe you twisted your back accidentally as you got out of bed—and that was the "straw that broke the camel's back."

My friend's daughter, Victoria M., teaches first grade and is always running after some child or playing with her students outside at recess. She often picks up a crying youngster or bends down to pick up something from the floor. In addition, she has two children of her own who keep her hopping. She is young and active but about 15 pounds overweight.

One weekday morning, Victoria was getting into her car to go to school when all of a sudden she felt a pang in her lower back. It nearly bent her in two, and she couldn't straighten up! She managed to hobble back into her house and lie down on her bed with a pillow under her knees. She called her school and said she wouldn't be in that day. Fortunately, she knew what to do for her back: She started alternating ice and heat for 5 minutes each for about half an hour. She swallowed some ibuprofen, an anti-inflammatory. And she made an appointment with her chiropractor and knew that she would need to take it easy for a few days, resting and moving gently as her muscles loosened up.

How Do You Know if Your Back Pain Is Minor or Serious?

If you suddenly develop pain in your back, especially your low back, where it is most common, try some of the remedies I'll recommend later (ice, moist heat, a nonsteroidal anti-inflammatory such as aspirin or ibuprofen). Take it easy for a couple days, although you don't necessarily need bed rest. In fact, experts now warn that bed rest longer than a couple days may weaken muscles and bones and actually slow your recovery.[3] For most people, the pain clears up or at least improves significantly within a few days. If it doesn't, you may want to consider a visit to your doctor or chiropractor. If you have any of the following symptoms, you may have a more serious problem, and you should talk with a doctor right away:

Symptoms of possible serious back-related illness

- ✦ Pain or tingling in your legs or extreme leg weakness
- ✦ Numbness in the groin or rectal area, legs, or feet
- ✦ Trouble controlling your bowels or bladder

A Quick Lesson on Back Talk

As you learn how to take care of your back and neck, here are some terms that will help you understand what's going on. (Refer to the diagrams of the spine.)

Vertebrae: the bones of the spine. The spine is identified by regions, with each region housing several vertebrae.

Discs: the cartilage that lies between the bones of the spine and lends cushion and structure to the spine. The discs are like sponges; they absorb shock and also keep the vertebrae separated and aligned.

Facet joints: load-bearing joints whose surfaces glide across one another, taking some pressure off the discs as they move. These joints control how far and in which direction you can move; many injuries result from overstretching a facet joint.

Herniated (slipped) disc: the protrusion, or bulging, of a disc into an area where it doesn't belong. One risk factor can be years of slumped sitting. Herniation is most common in the two lowest lumbar discs because they carry the greatest weight and are subject to the greatest range of motion.

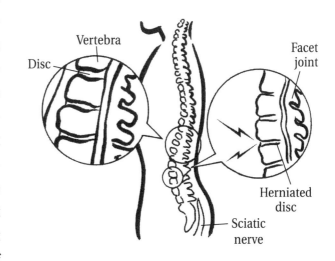

Spinal stenosis: a narrowing of the spinal canal, usually caused by degenerative changes in the spine. It most frequently affects people in their fifties and sixties, and it is twice as common in men as in women.

Sciatica: irritation of the sciatic nerve that runs down each leg. Often a result of a herniated disc or spinal stenosis, sciatica can resolve with little or no treatment within 4 to 6 weeks.[4]

Osteoporosis: a condition marked by fragile, weak bones caused by a loss of bone mass. It now affects 20 million Americans. Although both men and women are at risk as they age, the medical spotlight currently focuses on postmenopausal women who no longer have adequate levels of the hormone estrogen to prevent bone loss.

Spondylolysis: a stress fracture or weak area in the back portion of a vertebra, often the result of overstretching or hyperextending the back into an excessive arch. Athletes such as gymnasts, skaters, or long jumpers who arch their backs a lot are at greatest risk for this malady, but it can happen to anybody who overextends.

Curves of the Back

Your back has three natural curves. These curves add strength and flexibility to the back, and they absorb shock. The cervical curve is at your neck, the thoracic curve falls at your middle

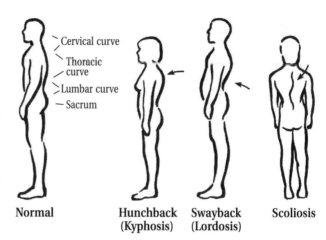

Cervical curve
Thoracic curve
Lumbar curve
Sacrum

Normal   Hunchback   Swayback   Scoliosis
                (Kyphosis)   (Lordosis)

back, and the lumbar curve covers the lower region of your back. Some experts consider the sacrum to be a curve as well; it comprises the fused vertebrae from the low back to your "tailbone." Usually, a painful back results from an imbalance among these curves, or what we commonly call "bad posture." Typically accompanying this imbalance are weak muscles, and tendons and ligaments that are tight and short from years of bad posture.

When the curves are exaggerated, three types of conditions can develop.

✦ *Exaggerated hunchback:* also referred to as kyphosis or dowager's hump. When it develops in adulthood, it is often caused by disc degeneration or osteoporosis.

✦ *Exaggerated swayback:* also known as lordosis. The abdomen is thrust too far forward and the buttocks too far back, a condition common in overweight people with weak abdominal muscles.

✦ *Scoliosis:* a common sideways deviation of the spine. Often congenital, it can be identified in childhood and prevented from getting worse. In adults, it can result from degenerative changes in the discs.

A well-aligned body preserves the natural curves of your spine, gives you good posture, and does not overuse one muscle group at the expense of others. Our mothers were right: Sit and stand up straight. Don't copy the military picture of ramrod-stiff posture, but strive for an erect spine with its natural, healthy curves supporting the rest of your body.

Categories and Causes of Back Pain

Sometimes it's easy to pinpoint the exact cause of back pain, but often there is no simple, obvious reason. You may be having your first experience with such pain, or you just may not be able to figure out how this could have happened to you. Here's how most back pain is classified and divided into categories.

Sprains, Strains, and Spasms: Muscle and Ligament Problems

Think of your muscles and ligaments as "guide wires" that support the spinal column. When muscles on one side of your body are too tight—improperly balanced against weak muscles on the other side—they throw the natural curves (cervical, thoracic, or lumbar) of your back out of proportion, and you can develop an ache just about anywhere. For example, if your thigh muscles (quadriceps) are too tight, that could lead to lordosis, too much of a curve in the lower back.

Sports medicine specialist Lewis G. Maharam, M.D., says in *A Healthy Back*[5] that back muscles are susceptible to injury primarily because they work so diligently and take so little time off. They're working even when you're standing or sitting still. And even if you are a "couch potato," a retiree, or a low-activity person, your muscles nevertheless need to be conditioned and flexible. Otherwise, it is possible to precipitate a strain or sprain with a motion as simple as reaching too far forward to open the refrigerator door!

As you can imagine, muscle and ligament problems are among the most common causes of back pain. Ligaments that support the spine can be sprained or torn. Muscles can be strained or

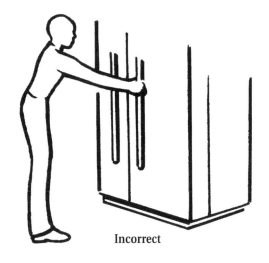

Incorrect

torn, or they can contract involuntarily in a spasm. Experts at Johns Hopkins University say that spasms, even though they can be excruciatingly painful, ultimately protect us because the pain ensures that the injured area will remain immobile, thus preventing further damage.[6]

Actions that may precipitate a muscle problem include overworking, bending or lifting something the wrong way, falling, twisting suddenly, or standing or sitting improperly. Even stress and anxiety can play a role because they cause muscles to tense up and possibly become more prone to injury.

Disc Problems

You could have some disc degeneration or herniation and not even know it. Only when you have symptoms, such as pain or stiffness, will you know that you need to investigate further. The most common site for herniation is the lumbar region. A herniated lumbar disc can cause pain, numbness, or weakness in one or both legs (sciatica). A problem with a cervical disc can result in similar symptoms in the arms or hands.

As you age, your body retains less water, so your discs dehydrate as well; they lose some of their shock-absorbing power. Discs also succumb to wear and tear as they help carry the heavy load of your torso. Over a long period of time, activities such as running with your feet pounding the pavement, or repeating rotational movements like a golf swing, can also stress and break down your discs.

Surprisingly, disc problems occur most frequently in the under-60 set. After age 60, your discs become less pliable and less mobile, and, therefore, they are less likely to protrude and cause trouble. However, this rigidity can lead to other problems of the spine.

Usually, a mild trauma, such as lifting an object or even sneezing, is enough to cause herniation of discs weakened by degenerative changes. According to researchers at Johns Hopkins, back pain that comes from a herniated disc pressing on a nerve root rarely requires surgery. They report that about 80 percent of patients with a herniated lumbar disc respond to treatment with some bed rest and pain medication, probably because the swelling around the nerve root subsides.[7] (Bed rest for a herniated disc may be more helpful than bed rest for a muscle or ligament problem. Check with your doctor.)

Miscellaneous Ailments

Back pain can also come from many other sources, such as

+ *Osteoporosis:* a condition of brittle bones.
+ *Rheumatoid arthritis:* an autoimmune disease in which the lining of the joints becomes inflamed.
+ *Osteoarthritis:* an illness involving chemical and structural changes in cartilage as well as hardening of the bone and formation of bony spurs around the joints.
+ *Leg length discrepancy:* a situation in which one leg is slightly longer than the other, usually easily corrected with foot orthotics.
+ *Vertebral compression fracture:* a condition that can occur from a violent injury (such as a car accident) or only a minor trauma (such as sneezing) if the vertebra is already weakened (from osteoporosis, for example).
+ *Cancer:* a disease sometimes found in the spine after it has spread from another place in the body.

Although you can always act to heal yourself, there are many instances when you need the partnership of the appropriate medical professional. As your doctor or therapist prescribes tests, medicine, or other treatments, you can add proper diet, exercise, and an optimistic attitude to enhance your health.

SUMMARY

Although millions of adults experience some type of back or neck pain, people are also learning more and more about how to prevent and alleviate it. If you get a kink in your back, a muscle spasm, or an unexplained pain, no longer do you have to go to bed for a week and hope it gets better. You can act to heal yourself.

Most back problems stem from today's frenzied lifestyles. You can prevent back pain (and other ailments) with

- Good posture
- Correct body mechanics
- Low-stress lifestyle
- Proper nutrition
- Regular exercise
- Support from your pillow and mattress
- Proper support wherever you sit or lie down

Now I'll go on to my favorite topic: getting you out of pain and then preventing it in the future.

How To Get Your Back On Its Feet *and* Prevent Future Pain

(Don't Skip This Chapter)

"People come to me and ask, 'Why me?
Why do I hurt?' I tell them pain is an indica-
tion they are doing something wrong."

JoAnne

HIGHLIGHTS OF THIS CHAPTER

✦ Self-treatment

✦ Ice and heat: contrast therapy

✦ Eleven paths to pain relief

✦ Importance of moderate exercise

✦ Motivation for good posture

✦ Proper body mechanics

✦ Advantages of stretching

✦ Hands-on body work for pain relief and healing

You might be the victim of an acute incident that has left you with a serious neck ache or backache. Or you may have chronic, annoying low back pain or a backache that comes and goes. Whatever your situation, many actions will bring you relief. You may have seen your doctor or a chiropractor. You may have ordered a new mattress or a new chair. Maybe right now the pain is virtually gone, or maybe it is still haunting you. Here are some immediate things you can do to relieve that pain and promote healing.

The latest thinking about sudden back pain has brought about bold changes in the way people treat such problems. No longer should you go to bed for 3 weeks or immediately run to the surgeon. In fact, up to 90 percent of people with a back injury recover within 6 weeks—without medical treatment and often with some self-treatment.[1] If ever there was an opportunity for self-healing, this is it. Many people relieve their pain with ice, heat, or both. (However, if severe pain persists, if you have symptoms such as pain or tingling in the legs, numbness, or trouble controlling your bowels or bladder, or if your pain does not respond to your own treatment, visit a doctor.)

Cold and Hot

Experts disagree on the use of ice and heat to treat back problems. Some say that you should use ice or cold packs exclusively during the first 48 hours after you feel the pain. I endorse "contrast therapy," the alternation of cold and heat for 5 minutes at a time for a total of about 25 minutes. Here's how it works:

> 5 minutes: ice or cold pack
> 5 minutes: heat or hot pack
> 5 minutes: ice or cold pack
> 5 minutes: heat or hot pack
> + <u>5 minutes: ice or cold pack</u>
> Total: 25 minutes

Take a break, then repeat the process several times a day. Of course, if your doctor or health professional recommends some other plan, please follow it.

Contrast therapy works because the cold reduces inflammation and the heat increases circulation to the area. Healing requires both.

To make this procedure easy, you can get a gel pack shaped to drape around

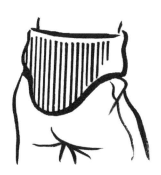 the area of your body that hurts, such as your neck, low back, or wrist. Keep the gel pack in the freezer, or heat it in the microwave. Most gel packs have Velcro® fasteners, so you can wear them as you go about your daily activities. Even easier to use are gel packs made with pockets for inserting either a cold or a hot pack. You can buy a few packs and alternate therapy without waiting a long time for a pack to refreeze.

When you do use heat to relieve pain, "moist" heat seems to work better than the traditional electric heating pad. A pack you heat in the microwave is considered to be moist heat. You can also stand in the shower with a wet towel over the area that hurts.

More Paths to Pain Relief

Here are some well-tested, safe actions you can take to relieve back pain. See what works for you.

✦ *Return to moderate activity and exercise, even if some discomfort is present.* Don't go back to your ear-splitting, foot-pounding aerobics step class right away. Don't bicycle 10 miles the day you finally start feeling better. It's fine to walk around, swim, and go about your everyday movements, though, as long as you can do them without major pain. As I've mentioned, bed rest for more than 36 hours may actually weaken your muscles and thus inhibit recovery.

✦ *Use over-the-counter analgesics instead of heavy-duty muscle relaxants that might make you drowsy.* The experts say that aspirin, acetaminophen (such as Tylenol™), or some other NSAID (nonsteroidal anti-inflammatory drug) such as ibuprofen can be just as effective in relieving pain as many prescription drugs, which are more expensive and sometimes have side effects.

✦ *Get your spine lined up properly.* Have an adjustment by a chiropractor or an osteopath who lines up your vertebrae as they were meant to be—taking the kinks out, in other words. In 1994, a respected medical panel appointed by the U.S. government gave official approval to the use of chiropractors and osteopaths for the relief of back pain.[2] That approval constituted a significant first. Of course, it didn't surprise those of us who know that these doctors have helped relieve suffering in millions of people with spinal problems.

> *"I was in a bad car accident, then hurt my back again when I moved to a new house. I had to wear a back brace every day. The back support cushion from JoAnne's is the first one that's ever worked for me. I also have one of your mattresses, and I use a wedge under my legs. It's amazing how each of these items takes the pressure off my back and makes me feel so much better."*
> —Rita Hecker
> Montgomery Village, Md.

✦ *Try a massage.* You may already have an electric or battery-powered massager that you can use on your sore spots. Or you can go to a professional massage therapist who knows how to find and ease tight muscles and ligaments. Or ask a family member or friend to massage you gently. There's nothing like having someone take care of you with a loving massage!

✦ *Use pillows or other supports.* Sleep with a pillow, knee wedge, or rolled-up towel under your knees to ease the pressure on your lower back. Try a neck support pillow or lumbar cushion that hits your body in just the right places to reinstate the proper curves to your spine.

✦ *Consider an adjustable bed.* You'll read more about adjustable beds in chapter 6, but I can't emphasize enough how soothing they are and how easy to use. When people first experience the support and relaxation that adjustable beds provide, they always say, "Why didn't I do this sooner?"

More Solutions

Here's a quick summary of other actions you can take to relieve back pain, particularly chronic or recurring pain. You'll run into these suggestions elsewhere in this book.

✦ Your feet should not dangle when you are sitting down. If you are short, get a collapsible footrest and carry it with you, like I do.

✦ Do some gentle stretching exercises to keep your muscles limber, but never do an exercise if it is painful. The "no pain, no gain" theory can prove damaging.

✦ Try walking, swimming, yoga, or other activities that restore and maintain a healthy body and soul.

✦ Remind yourself to be aware of good posture and body mechanics. Put notes in key places where you'll see them and heed them.

> *"Our anchor desk is high and we need to raise the chairs up to it, which was hurting the backs of my legs. With the footrest from JoAnne's, I'm much more comfortable. Many of our anchors use it; it's a lifesaver when we do long shows."*
> —Jane Karlen, Anchor,
> Newschannel 8
> Springfield, Va.

✦ De-stress yourself! Take steps to reduce or eliminate factors that cause stress in your life and tension in your body.

Moving On: Posture

Okay. You've eliminated most or all of the pain that ran your life for a few days or even longer. Or maybe you've never had a problem with your spine, but you're determined to avoid back and neck pain forever. There are many, many ways to strengthen your muscles and support your body's natural alignment. It should come as no surprise to you that spinal health starts with good posture.

When you were growing up, you may have been taught that having good posture meant standing stiffly "at attention." No! Good posture these days means allowing your body to maintain its gentle, *natural* curves of the spine.

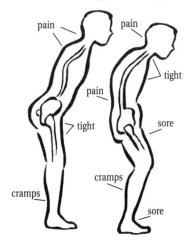

If you need any motivation to be aware of your posture, look at these drawings of the pain you could go through as a result of bad posture.[3]

If you look in the mirror and your body resembles either of these drawings, take heart—you can correct the situation. It may take a little time and some concerted effort, but it can be done, and you will feel a lot better.

For example, a common pattern of poor posture occurs with slouching and allowing the shoulders to roll forward into kyphosis. This distorted curve of the vertebrae in the upper back can shorten chest muscles over time and result in a round-shouldered look. Sometimes tall people stand this way in an attempt (either conscious or unconscious) to appear shorter. Here is a good way to stretch the chest muscles and correct even slight slouching:

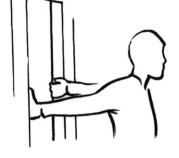

Stand in a doorway and hold both sides of it with your hands behind you at about shoulder level. Lean forward and straighten your arms. Keep your chest up and chin in. Hold for at least 30 seconds.

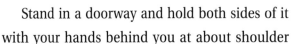

Dr. Nicholas DiNubile, special advisor to the President's Council on Physical Fitness and Sports, suggests a simple way to teach good posture to your muscles. Have someone stick a horizontal strip of tape on your back, stretching it from shoulder to shoulder. If you start to slouch, the tape will pull on your skin or shirt, reminding you to sit or stand up straight.[4]

All the Right Moves

Have you ever heard the term body mechanics? Mechanics is the aspect of science that deals with energy and forces. So body mechanics means the force and energy applied as you move your body. If this force is applied in the wrong way, overextending your muscles or overtaxing any part of your body, you could end up in pain.

As an example, consider what it takes to open a door. Ideally, you should step close to the door, a little less than arm's length in front of it. You should then place one foot in front of the other, bend slightly at the knees, keep your spine upright, and pull open the door. That's a lot to think about, isn't it? However, opening a door in this manner uses the strength of your legs and arms rather than straining your lower back by standing too far from the door and leaning too far forward to open it.

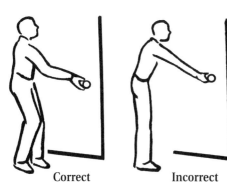

Correct   Incorrect

Think about how you bend down to pick up something or get something out of a low drawer or cabinet. If you bend at the waist with legs straight and reach out for the object, the strain goes onto your lower back. One study has found that people who lift improperly have twice the risk of a herniated disc compared to those who use the right technique.[5] To lift correctly, position your body close to the object, keep your back straight, and bend at the knees. Again, this technique lets you use your legs, which are often stronger than your back. Remember this advice when you pick up your child or grandchild, who keeps on getting heavier and heavier! Check these additional tips on how to use body mechanics to your best advantage:

Correct

- Don't plant your feet and overstretch your arms in an attempt to reach something; move as close as you can to the object, then reach for it.

- Get out of bed by rolling onto your side, pulling your legs toward your chest, then using your arms to support your weight while you simultaneously sit up and swing your legs to the floor.

- Get into bed from this sideways position also. Don't fall straight back from a sitting position.

- When you turn your head and neck to see something, turn your shoulders and upper torso as well. This puts less strain on your neck.

Now, if for some reason you *do* hurt yourself by overstretching, don't panic—it's probably only temporary. Use the contrast therapy I recommend: cold, then hot, on and off for the first day or two until the pain goes away. Ibuprofen, aspirin, or another anti-inflammatory aid may help. See your doctor if the pain persists and doesn't improve over a reasonable period of time.

The Goal of Fitness

As I told you in chapter 1, the Good Health Triangle includes exercise as an essential part of a healthy lifestyle. It's good for you and goes down a lot easier than castor oil. On top of that, most people who commit themselves to a regular exercise program actually start to enjoy it as they reap its benefits, which include

- Weight reduction
- Better emotional health
- Stress reduction
- More muscle, less fat
- Improved flexibility and strength
- Enhanced immunity
- Improved sexual function
- Increased bone density

Trainers classify exercise into three main categories: aerobic, strength training, and flexibility. When you pay attention to these three areas, you will gain the greatest benefits. Many people go on to work out for a specific sport or to concentrate in one area, such as weight training. But in general, if you divide your time among these three areas for a few hours each week, you'll be physically fit plus you'll have the right to be enormously pleased with yourself.

Since my main concern centers around helping you keep your spine in good shape, I want to concentrate here on stretching exercises.

First, I'll elaborate on the do's and don'ts of stretching that I mentioned in chapter 1:

✦ Always warm up your muscles a bit before you stretch; never stretch a cold muscle. Warm up with 5 to 10 minutes of aerobics or brisk activity.

✦ Pay close attention to being in the correct position when you stretch. Look at a diagram or go to a class until you learn the right way to do each stretch.

✦ Hold each stretch for at least 15 to 30 seconds while concentrating on sending breath into that area of your body so you can stretch as far as possible. It takes this long for the muscle to get the message that it's okay to relax and stretch.

✦ Never bounce in a stretch! Bouncing can tear muscles and tendons. Just relax into the stretch and hold it.

✦ Stop if you feel real pain. There's a difference between the satisfying feeling that you're doing a good job for your body and the pain of a tear or overexertion. Don't worry—you'll know the difference.

Let's Get Specific

Now, here are some diagrams of basic stretches that you can do every day to keep your spine supple and your body limber. For more details, I highly recommend the classic, well-illustrated book, *Stretching*, by Bob Anderson.

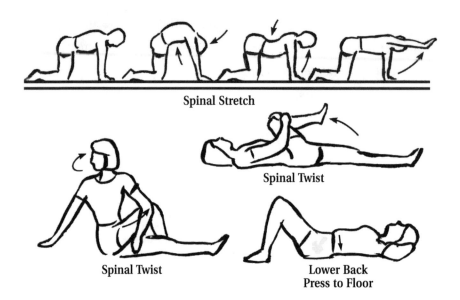

Spinal Stretch

Spinal Twist

Spinal Twist

Lower Back
Press to Floor

Body Work

Nope, I'm not referring to repairing that dent in your car door. I'm referring to the many kinds of therapy that can help you out of pain or can just help you relax and feel good. All these therapies and techniques honor what we now know about the clear connection between the mind and the body. These techniques also recognize the importance of the breath in releasing tension and sending healing energy throughout the body.

You don't have to wait until you're in pain to get the benefits of someone massaging you or working on you physically. Many people have massages regularly, as part of a "wellness" program or just to give themselves the gift of feeling good. Others may have significant physical problems that could be greatly relieved by a professional set of healing hands. Body work can relieve pain from

+ Whiplash
+ Pinched nerve
+ Arthritis
+ Osteoporosis
+ Multiple sclerosis

- Fibromyalgia
- Pain in low back, neck, hip
- Daily stress and tension
- Other ailments

I'll start with the type of body work that just about everyone has heard of: massage. When your spouse or a friend rubs your shoulders a bit after you've had a rough day, that's a form of massage. You may have had the benefit of a professional massage at a spa, a wellness center, or even at home. I'm a big fan of these treatments. As you investigate massages, you'll find there are many different types, including

- Swedish
- Deep-muscle
- Therapeutic
- Healing touch
- Shiatsu

Do whatever makes you feel good!

Other types of hands-on or awareness body work include

- Reiki
- Feldenkrais
- Rosen Method
- Rolfing
- Alexander Technique

I'll take just one, the Alexander Technique, to illustrate how you can help your body function better in this busy world.

Students of the Alexander Technique learn to expand their awareness of how they move in everyday actions, even those as simple as walking, sitting down, or standing up. It's a way of thinking about your movements and talking to your body so that muscle tension is dramatically reduced. Then when you do move, you move with great biomechanical efficiency and your muscles work only as much as they need to, not a bit more.

In Washington, D.C., certified Alexander teacher Lynn Brice Rosen says the technique not only helps people out of pain, but also helps prevent it down the road. "Our bodies are like delicately balanced mobiles," she explains. "Jumping up to answer the phone, for example, is a classic startle response, which activates a fight-or-flight reaction. Many physiological changes occur, and we overuse parts of the body, including muscles. This pushes other parts of the body out of shape in compensation. The Alexander Technique gives people the opportunity to choose how they respond to stimuli and return to an easy balance that supports the intended structure of the body."

SUMMARY

Back pain responds very well to simple treatments such as ice and heat packs (contrast therapy), over-the-counter pain relievers, and a return to moderate physical activity. If the pain persists, then you should see a doctor. A U.S. government panel has now approved the use of chiropractors and osteopaths for the relief of back pain. To feel better and prevent future pain, support your body with pillows and an adjustable bed, and seek out massages and other types of body work.

Good posture and proper body mechanics provide two of the most important ways you can take care of yourself. Stretching your basic muscle groups every day also makes a major contribution to your overall spinal health and flexibility.

Next, I'll cover more ways to care for your spine in one of the most important—and common—positions: sitting.

CHAPTER 4

Your Spine at Work, at Home, and on the Telephone

The Science of Ergonomic Seating

"Ergonomics—now, that's what I like. Shaping the environment to suit me and my needs is not selfish; it just brings greater satisfaction and productivity to my life."

JoAnne

HIGHLIGHTS OF THIS CHAPTER

✦ Ergonomics and the sandy beach

✦ Proper sitting position

✦ Support at work and in the car

✦ Ten tips for buying an office chair

✦ Loungers and recliners

✦ Seat lift chairs

✦ Telephone posture tips

✦ Care of your neck

Ergonomics and the Sandy Beach

In these high-tech times, people sometimes find themselves adjusting to or yielding to obstacles in their environment just because it's easier to "go with the flow." Yet this may be at the expense of their own comfort or safety, or because they feel they don't have any choices. Personally, I try not to compromise my standards; I like to have my environment adjust to me.

Ergonomics is the science of the environment adjusting to you, rather than you adjusting to the environment. I believe, for example, that instead of sitting in a chair that hurts your back or your legs, you should have a chair that adjusts to *your* body, to its uniqueness, so that nothing hurts. Instead of sleeping on a lumpy mattress, you deserve one that yields to your own body, yet gives enough firm support that you don't wake up with aches you never had before.

Think about going to the beach and lying in the sand. You wiggle around and make hills and valleys until the sand molds to your own body curves and makes you feel comfortable and relaxed, but solidly supported at the same time. Many chairs, recliners, beds, and pillows do that now, using modern construction and a unique material variously called visco foam, open-cell foam, or E-Foam™. This material is heat and weight sensitive, so as soon as you sit or lie on it, it starts molding to your unique body curves and angles. E-Foam™ is a fabulous technological advance; I can't praise it enough, nor can all the people I've introduced to it. More on this later.

Taking the Pressure Off

Do you ever wonder why your back can hurt more when you are sitting than when you are standing or walking? It's because there is more pressure on your lumbar discs when you sit. If you define the pressure when you stand as 100 percent, the pressure when you sit with a straight back becomes 140 percent. And when you sit leaning slightly forward, the pressure becomes 190 percent![1]

One of the best gifts you could give your back would be a well-designed chair for your office or your home, or a good back support for your car. Remember, ergonomics is fitting the environment to you—adjusting chairs and car seats to your unique body needs or using appropriate accessories. However, even with this kind of support, you need to be aware of several important factors when you sit.

How to Feel Comfortable When You Sit

Here's the correct body position for sitting at a desk, work station, or even the dinner table.

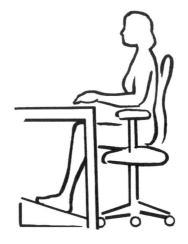

✦ Maintain the natural curves of your spine. Your low back needs to have that little lumbar curve and not be flattened against the back of the chair.

✦ Maintain alignment of your spine; don't slump.

✦ Sit all the way back in the chair.

✦ Keep your feet flat on the floor or on a footrest, or slightly angled up on a slanted footrest.

✦ Elevate your knees slightly above your pelvis, just short of a 90-degree angle.

✦ Check that your hips are at approximately a 90-degree angle with your back.

✦ Place your elbows at a 90-degree angle, at the same height as your working surface or table, with your shoulders relaxed.

✦ Keep your head upright and even with your shoulders.

✦ Think of your shoulder blades as sliding down toward your waist. This means keeping your shoulders straight, not hunched or rounded, with your chest in an open position.

If you are sitting in front of a computer terminal, follow these guidelines.

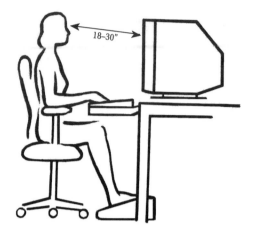

+ Keep your hands extended straight from your wrists, with wrists relaxed, not bent. Make sure the height of the armrests on your chair is about even with the computer table, not too high (causing you to scrunch your shoulders) or too low (causing you to bend your wrists too much).

+ Your line of vision should be even with the top third of the computer screen.

+ Your eyes should be about 18–30 inches from the screen. Relax them every so often by blinking and looking at something about 20 feet away.

+ Support your low back with your chair's built-in lumbar feature or with your own lumbar roll.

+ Position your document holder, if you have one, at the same height as the monitor and as close to it as possible. Also keep any other work tools close by, so you won't have to stretch far to reach anything.

+ Direct lighting away from the monitor, not onto it, thus eliminating glare.

When you are driving, use the position shown here.

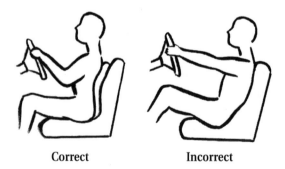

Correct   Incorrect

+ Sit close enough to the wheel for a comfortable reach, arms slightly bent and legs bent quite a bit.

+ Adjust the seat so your knees are slightly above the hips.

- ✦ Use a lumbar support or wedge if your back hurts.

- ✦ Move your hands frequently and keep them relaxed on the wheel.

Advice for Sitters

Regardless of where you are sitting, get up, stretch, and walk around at least once an hour. While you remain seated, teach yourself the habit of moving around slightly from time to time. Rotate your wrists and ankles; shrug your shoulders, then drop them into a relaxed position; turn your head gently; twist your torso; and do any kind of stretching or self-massaging that feels good and doesn't make you too self-conscious. If you are in the car, take a rest stop, get out of the car, and walk around.

> *"The back support and E-Foam cushion I bought for my car have given me tremendous relief. For the first time, I've been able to go on a long driving trip and not be bent over with pain when I get out of the car. It's really great."*
> —Bob Mulligan
> Washington, D.C.

What to Look for When Buying an Office Chair

The key to comfort in a desk or an office chair is adjustability. If you have a chair that doesn't adjust to the special needs of your body, you could waste a lot of productive time trying to get comfortable. A poorly designed chair can make even the ideal job feel like a torture session. A properly adjusted chair, on the other hand, helps maintain good posture, reduces back stress, facilitates relaxed arm placement for work, improves leg circulation, and minimizes fatigue. Ergonomics expert and physical therapist Marjorie Werrell says that having the correct chair is worth as many as 40 productive minutes to the work day. That's the time you save by not having to cope with neck, back, or shoulder pain from a poor-fitting chair.

Office chairs come in a wide variety of styles and prices: task chairs, computer chairs, managerial and executive chairs, and 24-hour intensive-use chairs. And don't worry—you don't need a pilot's license to operate modern office chairs. Your salesperson should have a full understanding of how each chair works and should demonstrate each one for you. You will quickly learn to move the basic levers that adjust the height, seat depth, tilt tension, and angles of your chair. Once these features are in place, just check them every once in a while to make sure they still support your body correctly. For example, to determine whether your seat depth is correct, you should be able to place a fist between the backs of your knees and the front of the seat. Of course, if you share the chair with someone whose size and shape differ from yours, you'll need to readjust the chair each time you use it.

The diagrams below have all the details about chair adjustability, but here are the basics you should know about.

- ✦ Tilt tension
- ✦ Seat height
- ✦ Seat depth
- ✦ Seat angle
- ✦ Back height
- ✦ Back angle
- ✦ Forward tilt and rock
- ✦ Arm height
- ✦ Arm width
- ✦ Seat and arm padding, preferably with ergonomic open-cell foam

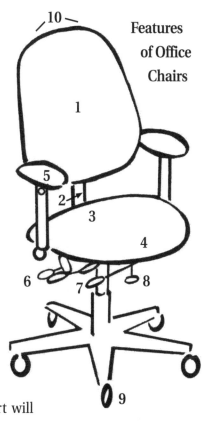

Features of Office Chairs

Features of Office Chairs

1. *Cradle yourself in comfort.* A contoured backrest with lumbar support will give your back the comfort and support it needs. Pick a chair shaped to match the natural contour of your spine.

2. ***Treat your back.*** Backrests that are height adjustable provide customized comfort and support.

3. ***Make the sit fit.*** For total comfort, seat and back foam must be dense enough to support your weight evenly and should be sculpted to fit the human form.

4. ***Go with the flow.*** Look for the "waterfall" seat cushions that slope down at the front of the chair. This important ergonomic feature helps improve circulation to your lower legs.

> *"My office chair from JoAnne's makes all the difference in the world. It used to be that I could sit only for a short time and the pain would start as soon as I stood up. Now I can sit as long as I want and my back won't act up. I'm very enthusiastic about this chair—I love it."*
>
> *—Jack Luria*
> *Potomac, Md.*

5. ***Arm yourself.*** Armrests help keep your arms in a comfortable position and thus reduce shoulder, neck, and back strain. The height adjustment knob is just below the armrest.

6. ***Please remain seated.*** Make sure all adjustment controls can be reached from a seated position.

7. ***Need a lift?*** The gas cylinder height adjustment mechanism lets you customize your seating position with a smooth, easy, one-handed action. Feet should be placed comfortably on the floor to reduce pressure on thighs.

8. ***Adjust to the job.*** Multi-tilt and articulating mechanisms are important for data entry or computer work. They let you vary your position while maintaining maximum support.

9. ***Roll right along.*** Good chairs have casters for easy mobility. Be sure to get the right kind for your floor or carpet.

10. ***Choose your weapon.*** Balance the features you require, the chair's design, and the quality of construction against your budget requirements before purchasing a chair.

Office Chair Operating Instructions

1. *Tilt Tension Control.* This knob controls the tension of the seat and the back tilting action. Turn the handwheel clockwise to increase tilt tension and counterclockwise to decrease tension.

2. *Pneumatic Seat Height Adjustment Control.* When you lift this paddle toward the seat and take your body weight off the seat, the seat goes up. When you lift the paddle while your weight remains on the seat, the seat returns to the lower position.

3. *Back Angle/Tilt Adjustment Control.* This paddle allows the back pitch to adjust at the front and back independently. When you pull the paddle up, the back angle tilts with your motion. When you push it down, the back angle locks into position.

4. *Multi-Tilt Control.* This paddle controls the infinite lock position. It locks the chair in any position you desire or allows the seat and back to float freely. To lock, push the paddle toward the floor. To free float, pull the paddle up.

5. *Back Height Adjustment Knob.* This control allows the back to adjust up and down. Turn the knob counterclockwise to loosen and slide the back either way. Once you have the position you want, turn the knob clockwise to lock it in place.

6. *Forward Tilt Lever.* This lever allows the chair to tilt forward. While you tilt the chair back slightly, rotate the lever toward the back or front. This action permits you to maintain maximum continuous tilt motion.

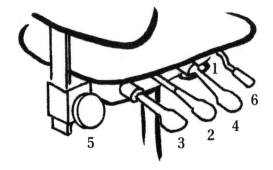

Chairs for Special Purposes

Kitchen and Dining Room

I know you want your kitchen and dining room chairs to look good as well as feel comfortable. I agree! But this doesn't mean they can't offer good support. When you buy new chairs, sit in them long enough to be confident that you will be comfortable for the duration of your meal. Make sure your spine is supported and you are sitting up straight. This posture helps you digest your food properly.

Loungers or Recliners

Just because you lie back and relax in a lounger or recliner doesn't mean your spine can't be aligned correctly. Some loungers come with built-in neck and lumbar supports, and sometimes you can add a small cervical pillow for your neck. Raising the "chaise" (leg) section of the lounger helps

Stress-Free Lounger

your circulation. In fact, a zero-gravity or stress-free lounger keeps your body in a position recommended by physicians: your hips, legs, and knees at almost 90 degree angles. This is how astronauts sit during lift-off.

Some recliners are constructed with tall people in mind and some are designed for shorter folks. Seat depth is an important factor. If you are short, you don't want a chair so deep that your legs dangle when you sit. Some loungers have heavy-duty frames and are built especially for people who weigh more than 300 pounds. When you shop, be sure that your body curves fit into the right places on the lounger and that it gives you all the features you want.

The ultimate pleasure, of course, is getting an automatic massage while you sit in your recliner. You can buy a portable insert that fits into any chair or even into the seat of your car; the insert starts massaging your back the instant you plug it in or turn it on. You can also treat yourself to a lounger that has built-in heat and massagers for the back and feet. The motors roll up and down on your gently warmed back as you relax in the chair. The heat and the massage increase circulation and therefore encourage healing in areas that may be achy or stiff.

Seat Lift Chairs

For people with arthritis, osteoporosis, or any condition that makes it difficult to sit down or get up, an electric seat lift chair is a blessing. With just the touch of a button on a hand control, the chair lifts you to a standing position so you can literally walk out of it. When you're ready to sit down again, you merely lean back against the chair and it takes you down to the sitting mode.

A less-recognized but excellent feature of a seat lift chair is that it doubles as an electric recliner. Once the chair has moved to its sitting position, you can use the hand control to recline to a resting, or in some chairs, a napping, position. For those who no longer have the arm or body strength to push themselves back in a manual recliner, this feature represents a dream come true.

Again, size counts. Don't put a small person in an oversized chair. Consider seat depth, seat width, and back height when you buy a seat lift chair.

Sitting and Your Neck

When you sit, the middle and lower parts of your back may not move around much, so it's relatively easy to adjust your chair or a lumbar support to keep those parts of your spine aligned. Your neck, however, might tell a different story. You might be twisting your neck to see something, angling it out of habit, or leaning forward to get closer to what you're looking at. For the sake of your neck, it's especially important to be conscious of good posture when you sit. And when you talk on the phone, your neck is at even greater risk of landing in a bad position. So now I want to go over some ways to protect your neck.

My 83-year-old mother-in-law, Henrietta, suffered from osteoporosis and nearly crippling back pain. She said she didn't want a seat lift chair, because it would be too costly and too complicated. But I insisted, and after a few days of using it, she couldn't imagine living without one. She would even relax in the chair at night when she couldn't sleep. The chair was sized to her short body, and she was delighted when the fabric blended perfectly with the rest of her furniture. It was a wise investment for Mom.

The Telephone: A Special Case

Most people can't exist without a telephone; some look like they have phones permanently attached to their ears. And many people try to accomplish other tasks as they chat on the phone. All this can build up to a tremendous amount of physical *and* emotional stress.

There are several ways you can alleviate the physical burden put on your muscles when you hold a phone.[2]

✦   A headset not only frees up your hands but also allows more normal movement of your head and neck as you talk. You can also use a speaker phone, especially for calls when you are listening more than talking or for calls when you are on hold for several minutes.

✦ Most right-handed people hold the phone with their left hand at their left ear; left-handed people do the opposite. Over time, these patterns can cause muscle imbalance that can lead to pain and injury. Try holding the phone to your right ear on even-numbered days and to your left ear on odd-numbered days.

✦ Move around while you talk on the phone. Stand up and stretch, or walk around if you have a cordless phone or one with a long cord. Even if you remain seated, shrug your shoulders, stretch your facial muscles by making funny faces with your jaws and eyes, or shake and lift your legs and arms.

✦ Massage yourself while you talk. Rub your neck and shoulders with your knuckles, fists, or fingers. Or use a massager such as the Jacknobber® to press on tight spots or acupressure points.

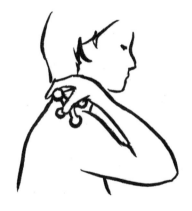

As for the mental or emotional stress that telephones add to daily life, remember that you can choose whether or not to answer that phone. If you're in the middle of something important, such as spending time with your family, enjoying a special meal, or doing some concentrated work—*just don't pick up the phone!* Rely on your answering machine or voice mail, or figure that if it's important enough, the caller will try again. Here's another way to cope with phone stress: train yourself to take a deep breath every time you hear the first ring, and wait until the second or third ring to answer. Conscious breathing adds a whole new dimension to getting rid of the stress in everyday life.

Easy Ways to Care for Your Neck

Ideally, of course, you pamper your neck and prevent any problems before they occur. Here are some of my favorite tips.

✦ Use a few spare moments each day to stretch your neck slowly and gently. Move your head up and down, and exaggerate the movement as if you were saying "yes." Then look side to side as if you were saying "no." Finally, tilt your head from shoulder to shoulder as if you were saying "maybe." Hold the end point of each position for a second or two, or longer if you want.

✦ If you work in front of a computer, look straight at the screen, with your line of sight extending to the top third of the screen. Sit at least 18 inches from the screen. Some new studies have found that the best distance from the screen is up to about 30 inches.[3]

✦ Sleep on a pillow that keeps your chin off your chest and aligns your spine. The pillow needs to fill in the empty space between the top of your back and the bottom of your head. (See illustration in chapter 2.) Keeping your vertebrae aligned also means refraining from sinking your head into a too-soft pillow, which could make your neck arch backward.

✦ *Never* prop a telephone between your head and shoulders—it hurts me to even think about this!

✦ Keep the rest of your body, particularly your spine, in good shape, with exercise, stretching, and proper eating.

SUMMARY

....

When you sit, you're putting tremendous pressure on your spine. Give it a break! Learn how to sit in proper alignment: your feet flat on the floor or on a footrest, your knees angled up slightly, your hips at approximately a 90 degree angle with your back, and your head upright and resting comfortably on your shoulders. Pay attention to your posture when you drive, when you work, when you dine, and even when you relax.

Necks often take a lot of abuse, and when they rebel, the pain can be truly awful. To prevent that pain, you need to be aware of how you hold your neck as you sit, work, and talk on the phone. You can care for your neck even when you sleep by using a supportive pillow.

Your spine will appreciate all this care, and it will repay you with pain-free days and good-sleep nights.

Speaking of nights, how do you get a good night's sleep in this crazy world of ours? Read on. I have some answers.

Oh, For A Good Night's Sleep

The Whys and Wherefores
of Restorative Rest

*"I can't emphasize enough the importance of a good
night's sleep, no matter how old you are. It can change
your whole view of life. And you can control just about
all the elements that make or break a good sleep."*

JoAnne

HIGHLIGHTS OF THIS CHAPTER

✦ America's sleep debt

✦ Your biological clock

✦ The role of melatonin

✦ Insomnia, snoring, sleep apnea,
and other sleep disorders

✦ Thirteen ways to improve your sleep

✦ Sleeping well during pregnancy

✦ List of information and support groups

Here's a stunning statistic: On any given night, one in three Americans has difficulty falling asleep or staying asleep.[1] According to the National Commission on Sleep Disorders Research, 40 million Americans suffer from chronic sleep disorders, and another 20 to 30 million individuals have intermittent sleep-related problems.[2] The commission warns that "America is severely sleep deprived." Many people are not even aware of the impact this deprivation has on their health and on their interactions with others.

For parents, young children can be the cause of not getting enough sleep. For women in mid-life, menopause and its symptoms may interrupt a good night's sleep. Teens can be anxious about anything from an exam to acne to a budding romance. Many senior citizens just don't sleep much at night for a variety of reasons, not necessarily the normal aging process. Even if you don't fit into one of these groups, sometimes you just might not get the ZZZs you want and need. Sleep loss accumulates from night to night (this is called sleep debt), so many people use the weekends to catch up.

Researchers in Australia have developed the Epworth Sleepiness Scale (right)

Are You Accumulating a Sleep Debt?

Rate your chances of dozing off in the following situations using the rating scale below:

3 = high chance of dozing off
2 = moderate chance
1 = slight chance
0 = none or stay wide awake

Sitting or reading	＿＿
Watching television	＿＿
Sitting in a public place (like a theater)	＿＿
Lying down for an afternoon rest	＿＿
Sitting or talking with someone	＿＿
Sitting down after a lunch without alcohol	＿＿
Being driven in a car for more than 1 hour	＿＿
Sitting in a car stopped in traffic	＿＿
Score	＿＿

If your total score is 0–5, you're probably getting enough rest. If your score is 6–12, you probably have a case of mild sleep deprivation. If you scored 13 or higher, you have chronic sleep deprivation.

to measure sleep deprivation in most people.[3] It asks you to look for everyday lifestyle clues to determine how you are affected by sleepiness.

According to the Better Sleep Council, average adults need between 7 and 8 hours of sleep each night. A handful can get by with 5 hours a night; another small group needs 10. Even more important than the amount of sleep you get is the *quality* of that sleep. Every night, you need deep, uninterrupted rest that consists of several distinct phases.

Stages of Sleep

In Stage 1, a twilight zone between full wakefulness and sleep, the brain produces irregular, rapid electrical waves. Your muscles relax and breathing becomes smooth and even.

In Stage 2, brain waves are larger and show occasional sudden bursts of electrical activity. You have now crossed the border between being awake and being truly asleep. If someone lifted your eyelids gently, you would not wake up.

In Stages 3 and 4, the brain produces even slower, larger waves, sometimes referred to as "delta" or slow-wave sleep. Your body functions, such as pulse, blood pressure, and temperature, are at their most lethargic. These four stages together are called quiet sleep, and they last for over an hour. This is where you get the most rest.

Then the brain shifts into a more active phase that is characterized by rapid eye movements (REM). This is REM sleep, and the earlier, four-stage phase is non-REM sleep. Vivid dreams occur during REM sleep, breathing is quick and shallow, and large muscles of the torso, arms, and legs cannot move, although the fingers and toes may twitch. Researchers believe REM sleep has mental benefits, including allowing learning and memory to gel.

During one night's sleep, adults spend about 75 percent of their time in non-REM sleep and 25 percent in REM sleep. Each cycle of non-REM plus REM sleep totals about 90 minutes, and adults experience four or five of these cycles a night. Normal sleep ends after a REM stage, which gives people that satisfied feeling of "a good night's rest." If the normal pattern of alternating stages is disturbed (by the jarring sound of an earlier-than-usual alarm clock, for example), sleep may not be fully restorative.

Different Strokes for Different Folks

The saying "sleep like a baby" may be a misnomer. Yes, babies do sleep soundly, but only for a few hours at a time. As people get older, their sleep patterns change dramatically; sleep tends to become lighter and more fragmented with the passing years. Yet some studies show that the need for sleep does not diminish much with age. As I've said, most adults need 7 to 8 hours a night on the average, no matter how old they are. Research also shows that about 30 percent of the population are natural "larks"—they enjoy being up quite early in the morning—and the rest of us are "owls"—we would rather bury our heads under the pillow than face the dawn.

Experts have arrived at the following generalizations about the amount of sleep people need.[4]

+ Full-term newborns: 18 hours a day
+ Toddlers and young children: 12 hours a day, some of it in naps
+ Kids from age 8 through late teens: $8^{1}/_{4}$ to $9^{1}/_{4}$ hours each night
+ Adults: Up to $8^{1}/_{4}$ hours a night

Sleep difficulties can occur at any age. One in every four children between the ages of 1 and 5 experiences some type of sleep disturbance such as nightmares, sleepwalking, or bedwetting. Teens tend to cut back on time in bed and suffer chronic daytime drowsiness as a result. For adults, the demands of job and family often subtract from the quality and quantity of sleep. (In a new survey, 57 percent of more than 1,600 U.S. workers report that they lost sleep because of workplace pressure.[5]) Menopause can trigger interrupted sleep. General insomnia and a breathing disruption called sleep apnea often develop in middle age. And by the time men and women reach their senior years, sleep patterns are so altered that they are often mistaken for part of the normal aging process. Yet these patterns are just forms of impaired sleep, many of which can be corrected.

I want to give you more information about sleep problems, and then we'll get to some solutions.

The Biological Clock Phenomenon

In his "Guide to Better Sleep, Everything You Need to Know From A—ZZZ's," Dr. Morton C. Orman discusses the changes in people's internal "biological clocks" as they age.[6] The part of the brain that controls sleep-wake cycles through the secretion of hormones creates "days" that are slightly more than 24 hours long. This is why it's easier for most people to go to bed late (since the body's sleep time is normally delayed) than it is to wake up early. In adolescence, a time of great hormonal changes, biological clocks often lengthen beyond 25 hours. Teens can stay up very late into the night but have trouble waking up at "normal" morning hours.

As people age, their internal biological clocks often shift to cycles lasting a bit less than 24 hours. So they tend to fall asleep earlier and wake up earlier. In turn, this might lead to more sleepiness during the day, more daytime naps, and the consequent inability to fall asleep at normal nighttime hours. Thus, older people don't really need less sleep—they just aren't getting enough. Their ability to sleep has been biologically impaired as a result of changes in their brain functions that are beyond their control.

The Role of Melatonin

The small pineal gland in your brain secretes the hormone melatonin in response to the dimming of light. Melatonin's basic purpose is to separate the body's daytime chemistries from its nighttime chemistries. It helps set those biological clocks. The brain synthesizes melatonin from another hormone, serotonin, which is made from the amino acid tryptophan. You can get tryptophan in your diet from eggs, cultured dairy foods, and beans. It is also found in turkey and milk. That's why your mom may have told you to drink a glass of warm milk before going to bed: for some people, it's a relaxant. Melatonin supplements have become very popular to overcome jet lag and to help people get to sleep at night, although its long-term safety has not been tested in rigorous scientific trials.

Scientists have determined that the brain of a young adolescent secretes its daily dose of melatonin at about 9:30 p.m., but in older teens, it occurs at about 10:30 p.m. This delays the entire night's sleep cycles, which may explain why older teens like to go to bed later and get up later. Some school districts are now experimenting with starting classes later in the morning, at 8:30 instead of 7:30, for example. These schools are finding that with the later starting time, students are more alert, ready to learn and participate, and less likely to have behavioral or disciplinary problems. Performance on exams has even improved.[7] Now you can understand everything that's going on with your teenager, right?

Sleep Disorders

With all this focus on sleep or the lack of it, I'd like to discuss the categories of sleep disorders. They range from merely annoying to potentially deadly. The information here only summarizes a vast field of research and information on sleep disorders. Treatments are available for most people with these difficulties; you'll find a list of resources at the end of this chapter.

Insomnia

Sometimes I have trouble sleeping and I'll get out of bed in the middle of the night to read or play a computer game. But it doesn't occur night after night. True insomnia is a lack of sleep so severe that it impairs your ability to function normally during the day. Most adults fall asleep within 30 minutes of getting into bed; people with insomnia often toss and turn for hours. Some wake frequently during the night or don't feel rested the next day, even if they have no apparent difficulty falling or staying asleep.

Anxiety and stress are the most common causes of temporary insomnia; clinical depression is often implicated in periods of insomnia that last a long time. Other factors associated with insomnia include poor sleep habits, physical symptoms (such as sore muscles or heartburn), arthritis, inappropriate medications, lack of exercise, and excessive use of alcohol or caffeine. As you might imagine, insomnia occurs often among shiftworkers.

With some determination, you really can master those sleepless nights. Treatments include learning relaxation techniques, restricting time in bed, improving sleep habits, and using sleeping pills on a short-term basis, perhaps to deal with a life crisis. I'll give you more detailed suggestions later in this chapter.

Snoring

About 25 percent of adults snore regularly and 45 percent snore at least occasionally.[8] Problem snoring is more frequent among men and also among overweight people, and it usually grows worse with age. Snoring occurs when there is an obstruction to the free flow of air through the passages at the back of the mouth and nose. As snorers sleep on their backs, the tongue falls backward, partially blocking the flow of air over the throat. Causes of snoring may include

- ✦ Tongue and throat with poor muscle tone.
- ✦ Throat tissue that is excessively bulky; for example, in children with large tonsils or overweight people who have bulky neck tissue.
- ✦ Deviated septum—a distortion in the wall that separates the nostrils.
- ✦ Stuffy nose due to a cold, sinus infection, or allergies.

Disturbed partners of snorers have come up with all sorts of solutions, from clips across the nose to surgical procedures to a good swift kick. If your partner snores, sometimes you just have to sigh and turn over. Believe me, I've done that myself. It's hard to say what will work for sure, although I know that if you snore, improving your sleep habits always helps.

Sleepwalking

About 2.5 percent of all adults sleepwalk regularly, and children between the ages of 5 and 12 are even more likely to leave their beds at night.[9]

Sleepwalking occurs during delta or slow-wave sleep, the deepest stage of dreamless sleep. It seems to run in families; children inherit a genetic tendency not only for sleepwalking but also for sleeptalking and bedwetting.

Leg Movements

Also known as Restless Legs Syndrome (RLS), leg movements affect about 5 percent of all adults and 10 percent of those over 65.[10] They feel a crawling, twitching, or pulling sensation in the legs while they are sitting or lying down and a nearly uncontrollable urge to get up and move around. The exact cause is still a mystery, but RLS appears to run in families and stem from a chemical imbalance in the brain. It also has been associated with rheumatoid arthritis, fibromyalgia, drugs for heart conditions and depression, and pregnancy. In a related disorder, the legs jerk violently during sleep, often enough to wake you up. Treatments include regular exercise (including a walk before bedtime), stretching, relaxation therapies, hot baths, cold compresses, massage, and some drugs.

Sleep Apnea

In Greek, apnea means "no breath," and that's exactly what happens. People with apnea stop breathing for 10- to 60-second periods dozens of times during the night. This disorder affects an estimated 18 million North Americans, and its prevalence increases with age.[11] One possible symptom adds ear-splitting snores to the pauses in breathing. Of course, waking up so much during the night produces excessive daytime sleepiness and a compromised quality of life.

As you can imagine, this is a serious problem. In most cases, apnea occurs when an obstruction in the airway, such as flabby throat muscles or a large tongue, temporarily blocks the flow of air to the lungs. Obesity, chronic nasal congestion, smoking, and excessive alcohol use can make the condition worse.

Apnea can contribute to potentially fatal problems such as high blood pressure, heart disease, and stroke. Weight loss provides relief in overweight individuals. Other treatments include a surgical procedure to enlarge the airway and a device that pushes a constant flow of air through a nose mask while you sleep.

A friend of mine, Amy S., went to her dentist. He told her that nighttime bruxing had worn her teeth almost flat. The dentist made a nightguard for her. It's a plastic appliance shaped to your upper teeth, so when you bite down unconsciously during the night, you won't wear away your teeth—you will just bite on the plastic. At her next checkup, the dentist informed Amy that the nightguard had halted the wearing away of her teeth, and she was able to tell the dentist she no longer woke up with headaches.

Bruxism (Teeth Gnashing)

More than 20 percent of adults and children grind their teeth at night! Sometimes a trip to the dentist helps; sometimes you need to have a discussion with your mind. Here's a surprisingly simple technique to stop grinding that may help you: Clench your teeth firmly for about 5 seconds, then relax for 5. Repeat 4 to 6 times a day.

In one study, 75 percent of bruxists stopped after 21 days of this self-treatment!

Narcolepsy

An estimated one in every thousand people has this disabling neurological disorder of the brain's sleep-wake control mechanisms, but those who are afflicted often don't know they have it. Regardless of how much narcoleptics sleep at night, they cannot stay awake during the day. They doze off, even while eating, talking, or driving. They can develop nighttime symptoms as well, including muscle problems.

Narcolepsy may be hereditary, and treatments include good sleep habits, daytime naps, and stimulant medications to control sleepiness and muscle weakness during the day. As yet, there is no known cure.

Physical and Environmental Causes of Poor Sleep

Studies show that most of the time when your body moves as you sleep, your sleep becomes more shallow. That is, the quality of your sleep suffers, and you may wake up sooner. Many factors, such as light, sound, temperature, or your partner's movement, can cause your body to move, but the less you move, the deeper your sleep will be.

The hardness of your mattress may also be a factor in how much you move around at night. According to ergonomics researcher Robert Oexman, people do have a tendency to move more on a harder surface.[13] As you will read in chapter 6, mattress surfaces should not feel *hard*—they should feel *firm, yet comfortable*. A comfortable mattress can give you all the support you need. I always say you should be kind to your body and give it that plush feeling. This, in turn, will lead to deeper sleep.

Consequences of Not Getting Enough Sleep

As I've said, the experts call lack of sleep a sleep debt or sleep deprivation. Stanford University professor Dr. William Dement, chairman of the National Commission on Sleep Disorders Research, warns that sleep debt is "potentially the most costly problem to our society in terms of dollars and human suffering."[14] The commission estimates that sleep disorders and sleep deprivation cost the United States almost $16 billion a year in direct costs and as much as $150 billion if you add lost productivity. Moreover, the commission claims that the NASA Shuttle's Challenger disaster, the Exxon Valdez oil spill, and numerous air, rail, and road accidents all could have been avoided if the people involved had been getting enough sleep.[15]

Scientists have documented these consequences of sleep deficit:

✦ Slowed reaction time, leading to train and traffic accidents or other workplace mishaps

✦ Lack of energy

✦ Daytime drowsiness, yawning, nodding off

- ✦ Irritability, emotional instability, and depression
- ✦ Less creativity (the kind needed for problem-solving)
- ✦ Less spontaneity
- ✦ Mistakes in everyday chores
- ✦ Stress

How to Improve Your Sleep

A pill isn't necessarily the answer. Whether it's a prescription from your doctor or an over-the-counter aid, it may mask the real cause of your insomnia. In fact, some of the *consequences* of inadequate sleep I listed earlier, such as stress or depression, may also be the *causes* of poor sleep. Before you run to the medicine cabinet for a solution, take some time to ask yourself what the real problem might be. Then, take steps to solve it, and consider these non-medical alternatives:

- ✦ *Catch up on your sleep.* It's as simple as that. For several nights, just allow yourself to sleep as long as you want until you wake up feeling rested. Most people recover after two such nights. You will then be at the natural level of sleep that you need. Promise yourself you will get that amount of sleep as much as humanly possible.

- ✦ *Go for quality sleep, not quantity.* Six hours of good solid sleep can make you feel more rested than 8 hours of light or disturbed sleep. Don't set a rigid rule that you have to get 8 hours sleep a night—let your body tell you what it needs. Some people need only 5 to 6 hours, others need 9 to 10.

- ✦ *Exercise regularly.* Make sure you are getting enough exercise during the day to allow your body to relax at night. Many studies show that regular aerobic exercise improves sleep. However, don't exercise late in the evening just before bedtime. Doing this could overstimulate you. For many folks, the optimum time to exercise is in the late afternoon or early evening before dinner. Exercising at this time releases the stresses of the day and relaxes you for the evening ahead.

+ ***Reduce stress.*** Spend time on yourself, use relaxation techniques, and try to achieve that elusive balance among all the people and tasks that vie for your attention. I find that when I take time for myself, whether it's lunching with a friend or curling up with a good book, I'm much better able to meet the demands of my job and my family. (See chapter 9 for more on stress management.)

+ ***Discipline the mind.*** If your mind won't quit even when you go to bed, try setting aside half an hour early in the evening to concentrate on issues and problems. Write down possible solutions, and tell yourself that you will resume dealing with those issues tomorrow.

+ ***Practice good sleep habits.*** Sleep in a totally dark room (light stimulates the brain into wakefulness). An excessively warm room disturbs sleep, but there is no evidence that an excessively cold room helps you sleep better.[16] Try to retire and awaken at about the same time each day, and sleep no more than you need to feel refreshed and vital.

+ ***Establish a relaxing bedtime ritual.*** Put a definitive end to the business of your day and turn to quiet activities that attract you, such as listening to music, reading, writing in a journal, or stretching and relaxing your muscles.

+ ***Don't go to bed stuffed or starved.*** Digesting food, especially high protein or high fat food, takes energy and forces the body to concentrate on digestion rather than relaxation. You want all your internal systems to slow down at bedtime, not speed up. On the other hand, if your stomach is rumbling from hunger, that could keep you awake as well. A light, low-calorie snack such as a piece of fruit or toast will help you settle down. Some people drink warm milk, which contains the amino acid tryptophan, a relaxant. Herbal teas with chamomile or valerian root also may help you relax.

+ ***Avoid sleep-disturbing drugs such as caffeine, nicotine, and alcohol.*** Some people swear that a glass of wine helps them fall asleep. Yes, it may do that, but alcohol can have a rebound effect that interrupts deep sleep and wakes you a few hours later. And for most people, caffeine and tobacco make falling asleep more difficult.

✦ *Check with your doctor about when to take medications.* Drugs such as beta blockers, antidepressants, decongestants, and steroids may have special times of the day when they are most effective. Follow your doctor's instructions or package directions on an over-the-counter medication.

✦ *Sleep on your back or your side.* Many people sleep on their stomachs, but as medical professionals will tell you, this does not support your spine. Sleeping on your stomach increases the lumbar lordosis (improper curve in your lower back) and places too much strain on your neck. You may think you can't sleep any other way, but sleeping on your stomach could get you into trouble. I can't emphasize this too strongly:

Never sleep on your stomach!

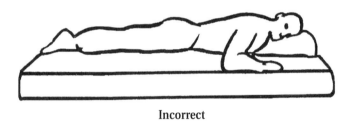

Incorrect

✦ **Try a new pillow.** Pillows wear out even more quickly than mattresses. You will be surprised and delighted with the difference a new pillow can make. When you sleep, your chin should be off your chest (not tucked down into your chest) and your spine should be aligned, with its natural curves in place all the way up through the neck. A pillow built with a comfortable "roll" under the cervical

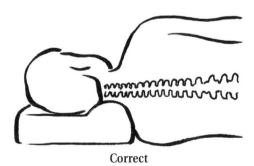

Correct

vertebrae provides proper neck support. Try a pillow made from open-cell foam, the ergonomic material that softens just the right amount as it "reads" your body's temperature and weight. I promise, you'll love it!

✦ *Do an annual bed check.* When you think you have a sleep problem, you may actually have a bed problem. It may be time for a new one. After about 10 years of nightly use, even the best quality beds may need to be replaced. See chapter 6 for a list of questions to determine whether you need a new bed.

> *"The first morning after the mattress was delivered, I got out of bed without lower back pain for the first time in years. I have been doing the orthopedic exercises for the lower back for more than 20 years. I am continuing with them, but they are much less 'challenging.' Also, I have slept better since the new mattress was delivered.*
>
> *"Your organization is most helpful to those of us who have back problems. Recent publications have documented how many of us there are."*
>
> —Bill Chapman
> Hillsdale, N.J.

Pregnancy: A Special Time

Mothers-to-be cherish their sleep as they wait for the time when they know their rest will be interrupted every few hours. Besides, most pregnant women tire more easily than before they became pregnant, and they need more sleep, both in naps and during the night.

As the belly grows larger and larger, finding a comfortable new sleeping position, while possible, can be a bit difficult. The best time to train your body for those new positions is early in the pregnancy. For obvious reasons, you won't be able to sleep on your stomach. And the experts say you should give up sleeping on your back, because you would be putting on your spine the entire weight of your uterus, intestines, and the vein that carries blood from the lower body to the heart.[17] So that leaves your sides—and preferably your left side—to allow better circulation.

Curl up on your side and put a pillow between your legs. This allows maximum flow of blood and nutrients to the placenta and enhances kidney function, which means better elimination and less swelling of your ankles, hands, and feet. Don't worry, however, if you wake up and find yourself on your back or belly. Most people don't stay in one position the entire night. Just turn back onto your side and snooze away.

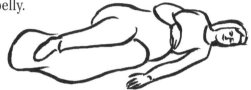

My niece, Karen, is expecting her first child. She's having a picture-perfect pregnancy but does find that she tires very easily and appreciates naps and going to bed early. She has a unique L-shaped pillow that she wedges between her legs as she sleeps. After the baby is born, Karen will lean up against this pillow for arm, back, and shoulder support when she feeds the baby. Then when the baby can hold her head up, Karen will nestle the baby into the two "arms" of the pillow and use its fabric ties to keep the baby upright.

SUMMARY

If you are dissatisfied about any aspect of your sleep, remember that you are not alone. Millions of Americans have sleep problems, and if you are one of them, you definitely have the power to do something about it. Most sleep disturbances are temporary, and when you focus on changing your habits, you can significantly improve your sleep and therefore your overall health.

Some of the suggestions I've made include these:

+ Sleep enough hours until you feel rested.
+ If your mind races when you try to fall asleep, set aside time earlier in the evening to focus on concerns and problems. Then, set them aside until the next day.
+ Sleep in a totally dark room.
+ Keep the room temperature moderate—not too warm, not freezing cold.
+ Exercise regularly but not right before bedtime.
+ Establish a bedtime routine that helps you relax.
+ Avoid caffeine, nicotine, and alcohol at bedtime.
+ Make sure your mattress and pillow support you well.
+ Never sleep on your stomach.

Now that you know how to get all the rest and good sleep you need, it's time to learn how to buy a new mattress and get the best possible value and quality.

Information and Support Groups
for Sleep and Sleep Problems

American Sleep Apnea Asssociation
1424 K St., NW, Suite 302
Washington, DC 20005
(202) 293-3650

American Academy of Sleep Medicine
6301 Bandel Rd., NW, Suite 101
Rochester, MN 55901
(507) 287-6006

Canadian Sleep Society
c/o Dr. Alistair Maclean
Psychology Department
Queen's University
Kingston, Ontario, K7L 3N6
(613) 545-2480

National Sleep Foundation
1522 K St., NW, Suite 500
Washington, DC 20005
(202) 347-3471

How to Buy a Mattress or a Whole New Bed

Ask Yourself "The Dozing Dozen"

"We spend about one-third of our life in bed. Let's say you're 60 years old. If you have a bad mattress and you don't get a good night's sleep, that's the same as 20 years—days, nights, weekends, and holidays—of tossing, turning, and morning grumpiness!"

JoAnne

HIGHLIGHTS OF THIS CHAPTER

- ✦ Deciding whether it's time
- ✦ Mattress lingo
- ✦ Hard vs. firm
- ✦ Coil count
- ✦ Price and warranties
- ✦ Mattress care
- ✦ Extreme comfort: E-Foam™
- ✦ The ultimate treat: adjustable beds

Mattresses wear and deteriorate very slowly—so slowly that your body starts accommodating to the mattress, rather than the mattress adjusting to your body. This is the opposite of ergonomics! That's why a mattress may need to be replaced approximately every 10 years, even if it doesn't look worn down. It depends on several factors, including the original quality of the mattress, whether it's been used every night, and whether it's been cared for properly.

I can't emphasize enough the importance of having a mattress that supports your spine. A mattress should fit like a shoe—comfortable, but with good support. You can guarantee that support by shopping at a store where you are confident that *all* the mattresses meet high quality standards, even the lower-priced options. Once there, test different models and buy what feels best.

Deciding Whether It's Time

Here's a list of questions you can ask yourself to determine whether you need a new mattress.[1]

1. How does the cover look? Is it torn or excessively soiled?
2. Does the mattress surface or the boxspring sag or look uneven?
3. Do you wake up feeling achy or stiff?
4. Is the mattress comfortable in some places and in some positions, but not in others?
5. When you turn over, do you hear creaks or other noises?
6. When you roll around, does the bed quiver or sway?
7. Are you and your partner unintentionally rolling together?
8. Are you fighting each other or thrashing with the covers for enough room to get comfortable?
9. Have you been sleeping on the same bed for many years and find that you don't feel as rested in the mornings as you would like?

Let's say the ache in your back prompts you to buy a new mattress and you've seen lots of ads with enticing deals. Maybe your doctor has told you to get a "firm" mattress to help your back. Or maybe you've considered the questions above and are convinced you need a new bed, but you just don't know how to go about making it happen.

Well, I will award you a "Ph.D. in Mattressology" after you read the rest of this chapter. First, some basic terminology.

- ✦ *Mattress:* the thick pad you lie on. It is made with a core of innersprings or foam covered with various layers of padding (e.g., cotton, polyurethane foam, fiber pads, dacron, latex, wool, silk, or open-cell foam). The mattress is finished by enclosing the entire package in a cloth ticking material. Mattresses come in twin, full (double), queen, or king widths and also as twin or full extra long. See the chart on the next page.

- ✦ *Boxspring:* supports the mattress. As much as 40 percent of your body's impact on a mattress is absorbed by the boxspring. A typical construction consists of a wood frame with metal coils attached to it, then a metal grid atop the coils, then a layer of padding, and finally, a cloth cover with ticking on the sides.

- ✦ *Foundation:* a boxspring made only of wood and foam. It is also covered by cloth with ticking on the sides.

- ✦ *Mattress set:* mattress plus boxspring or foundation.

- ✦ *Bed frame:* supports the mattress and boxspring or foundation, raising the top of the mattress to standard height. (This amounts to about 23 inches, but it can be more or less depending on the thickness of the mattress.) The frame is made of angle iron and is normally placed on casters. For king and queen mattress sets, the frame must have a center support. In fact, manufacturers' mattress warranties state that they are void for kings and queens if the frame does not have a center support.

- ✦ *Adjustable bed:* a bed that can be adjusted to bend under the knees and at the

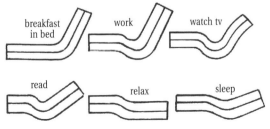

breakfast in bed   work   watch tv

read   relax   sleep

upper back. Using a hand control, you can raise and lower the bed at those points, changing positions to maximize comfort and proper support.

✦ *Open-cell foam or E-Foam™:* also known as visco, Swedish, or memory foam. I call it the Ergonomic Miracle. It's a material that yields, yet conforms, and supports every part of your body that rests on it. More below.

✦ *Topper:* a thick mattress pad, often made of E-Foam, convoluted polyurethane foam, or latex foam.

MATTRESS SIZES	
Twin	39" x 75"
Twin extra long	39" x 80"
Full	54" x 75"
Full extra long	54" x 80"
Queen	60" x 80"
King	78" x 80"
California King	72" x 84"

"The Dozing Dozen"

Now that you know the basics, here are 12 questions and answers to help you as you shop for a new mattress or bed.

What mattress are you sleeping on now?

Is it innerspring or foam? If it's foam, is it latex or polyurethane? Is it a waterbed or an air mattress?

You may have acquired your bed from someone else in the family, or you may be sleeping in the bed you've had all your life, or you may have bought the bed a long time ago. In any of these circumstances, you may not know the history, type, or origins of the bed. But it is valuable if you can find out because you will be able to make a more informed decision as you buy your next mattress.

I don't recommend water or air beds because I believe they do not support your head and neck properly. They have nothing to help you maintain the natural curves of your spine. If you do sleep on a water or air bed, try switching to innerspring or foam. If you already have an innerspring or foam mattress, stick with it. It's what you are used to and what you will probably find to be the most comfortable.

What size mattress do you want?

I suggest all couples buy at least a queen-size if not a king-size mattress set. You will find the extra room helps you both get a better night's sleep because you are less likely to disturb each other as you shift around. Also, if you are tall, a longer-than-usual 80-inch bed might allow you to sleep without your feet dangling off the end—perhaps for the first time since you were a kid. (The standard length for all the adjustable beds that my stores sell is 80 inches. I can also order just about any other mattress in an 80-inch length.) Measure the space you have available in your bedroom, and fit in the largest bed possible.

Besides getting a good night's sleep, do you have a specific use or health need that your new bed must satisfy?

My uncle developed severe sciatica pain in his low back and right leg, and he wanted an adjustable bed so he could find a position that relieved the pain. You might have a hiatal hernia or circulation problem that requires head or leg elevation. Adjustable beds also bring great relief to people with respiratory problems. Or perhaps you just like to read or watch TV in bed. Adjustable beds provide perfect solutions to these needs.

If you have arthritis, pay particular attention to the surface of your new bed to make it as comfortable as possible. You can get an E-Foam mattress or an E-Foam topper for your current mattress that provides proper support while giving relief at the pressure points or aching parts of your body.

What "feel" do you want in your mattress?

This is the most important quality of a mattress, but most people misunderstand what to look for. Many people think they need a "hard" mattress to support their backs, but let me tell you—*hard is not good!* I've learned this over my many years of helping people get a good night's sleep. Whether or not you have a back problem, what you really need is support and comfort at the same time. I call this the "feel" of the mattress, and the appropriate word to describe the feel you want is "firm," not "hard."

As *New York Times* writer William Hamilton puts it, "A mattress is going to be your worst enemy or your most important friend."[2] As you sleep, your spine (including your neck) should be in alignment. So when your body shifts positions during the night, your sleeping surface needs to be flexible as well, to preserve spinal alignment. If the surface is too hard, it won't be able to support your body at key points like the hips and shoulders. If the surface is too soft, your body will sag into it.

The least expensive mattresses are actually the hardest, because they consist of only springs with a little padding. Of course, springs are important for a foundation of good support, but padding is crucial for comfort. Ergonomics consultant Dr. John J. Kella says, "Padding relaxes the muscles and helps the body avoid pressure points. If the mattress is too firm, you'll tense up."[3]

Think back to that important concept, ergonomics. The mattress needs to conform to your body; your body has no obligation to adjust to the mattress. When you lie down, your entire body, mind, and soul should have the experience: "This is it. This is what rest is all about."

What about coil count and coil design?

This is confusing stuff! You may hear many different claims about coil systems, but according to *Consumer Reports*, "Neither coil design nor coil count affects quality or durability in all but the cheapest mattresses."[4] *Consumer Reports* adds that various spring configurations may feel slightly different when you're sitting on a mattress, but not when you're lying down. So don't let any salespeople try to sway you by emphasizing coil count; tell them you have other criteria for finding the right mattress set for you.

What about the fabric covering (the ticking)?

Since you're going to cover the fabric with linens, a blanket, and probably a spread or quilt, don't worry much about how pretty the fabric looks. On the other hand, fabrics do create different feelings as you lie on them, because they have different "gives" or resiliences. A knit, for example, gives or yields much more than a damask due to the tightness of the weave. The more cotton a fabric has, the more it "breathes" and the less it retains odors. The fabric contributes about 20 percent of the overall feel that you'll be evaluating as you test different mattresses in the store.

What about the filler material?

This too affects the feel of your mattress. You might ask, "Why care what filler is used as long as I get the overall feel I want?" Well, you need to pay some attention to this, because some fillers remain naturally resilient over a long period of time, and some compress more quickly. Garnetted cotton, the material in those thick wads that provide a lot of the puffiness in some mattresses, tends to compress and lose resilience. Polyester batting doesn't hold up as well as polyurethane foam. And polyurethane foam doesn't measure up to the new open-cell memory foam (E-Foam). As you shop, ask about what's creating the feel you like, so you can be sure it will be with you for the life of the mattress.

Do I need a new boxspring or foundation?

In general, yes. Boxsprings and foundations wear down over time, just as mattresses do, although you don't always know it because you don't lie on them directly. And remember, since "feel" is what you're after, you should buy the same system—the mattress and foundation set—that you tried and liked in the store.

Incidentally, make sure you have a good frame for your new bed (with a center support if it is a queen or king). Believe it or not, the quality of bed frames varies widely; some give much better support than others.

Now, the big question for many folks: What about price?

Beware of $99 or $118 or any other cheap specials. Such mattresses are poorly constructed and may end up hurting you more than helping you. Nor do you have to spend $2,500 for a mattress set. Many excellent beds are available in the mid price range: queen sets from $599 to $1,699; kings from $799 to $1,899. They will give you proper support and allow you the full benefit of a relaxing, pain-free night's sleep. After all, that's what you want, right?

Adjustable beds are obviously more expensive because they have motors, controls, and mechanisms to make the bed move up and down. However, I truly believe they are well worth the price. As the population ages and more and more people have back trouble, I think adjustable beds offer a pain-free lifestyle that can't be beat.

With all this information gathering and shopping, you may be overwhelmed and tempted to put a quick fix, such as a plywood board or egg-crate foam topper, into your poorly performing old bed. Please resist the temptation! Ergonomics consultant John Kella tells people to start fresh with a new bed. If you try to save what you would spend on a new mattress, he says, you'll spend much more than that at the doctor's office.[5] I agree. Cheaper is not better. Buy your new bed based on all the other factors you've learned about here.

> *Adjustable beds are handy for temporary problems, too. When my son, Mark, broke his right ankle, he had a lot of pain in his left leg, because he was putting so much more weight on it than usual as he hopped around and used his crutches. Elevating both his legs in an adjustable bed really helped alleviate the pain.*

How important is the warranty?

The warranty does not tell you how long to keep your new mattress and foundation; it's there to protect against product defects. Your bed may still be in one piece after 15 to 20 years, but it's probably not giving the optimal support you deserve. Its useful life, as I've said, is really about 10 years.

Note that the warranty is a manufacturer's warranty, not a store warranty. Each part of the product may be covered separately. Be sure to retain your receipt showing the date of purchase, and keep warranty information in a safe place.

How will I truly know it's the right mattress for me?

Trust your judgment! Since the ultimate test of a mattress is your personal preference, you need to test it at the store when you have plenty of time. Lie on the mattress on your back and on each side. Use a comfortable pillow, even your own if you want to bring it from home. If you read in bed, prop yourself up as if reading a book and see how that feels. Don't be embarrassed; salespeople expect you to give it a trial run (clothes on, of course). Merely sitting on the edge of the bed won't give you an idea of the feel either. Lie down, and let the salesperson see how the mattress fits you. If your back happens to hurt a little the day you go shopping, try the mattress that day, then come back another time to test the mattress under more "normal" conditions.

A good mattress and foundation supports your body gen-

> "We purchased a new 'Spine-Align,' 'split top' premium queen mattress for our adjustable bed. Our original mattress seemed to be too soft and spongy, possibly contributing to back, leg, and hip pains experienced by both of us.
>
> "Difficult as it is to test a mattress in a showroom, you assured us that the firmer Spine-Align would help our condition. You were accurate … we have been most pleased with the results. My wife no longer complains of hip and leg pain. My back condition has also reflected measurable improvement … and we are sleeping better!"
>
> —Jack I. Hamlin
> Arlington, Va.

tly at all points and keeps your spine in the same shape as a person with good standing posture. With too little support, you may develop back, neck, or leg pain; too rigid a mattress may make you experience uncomfortable pressure.

Your mattress should fill in the curves of your body, in the lumbar area, thighs, calves, and shoulders. As people age, they have different needs; they still need good support, but they may want more surface softness. Remember, be kinder to your body as you grow older. You want an ergonomic relationship with your mattress, one where the mattress conforms to, supports, and accommodates you, not the other way around.

"We bought a queen-size bed, just perfect for our needs. We were the couple recommended by the chiropractor, if you remember. Just to let you know: we now both finally sleep all night and are extremely comfortable. We never thought we would ever sleep like that again. In our old bed, it would take at least 2 hours to fall asleep; with this new one we get drowsy in 10 minutes or less. Our bed is the best buy we ever made."
—Mr. and Mrs. Andrew Blanc
Westbury, N.Y.

Also, some retailers promise a "comfort guarantee" that allows you to exchange a mattress if you are unhappy after you try it at home. Terms for exchange vary, but the typical tryout period runs between 14 and 30 days, and there are generally some costs you may have to pay. Ask about this when you make your purchase.

Your new bed or mattress may remind you of a new pair of shoes: both require some time to "break in." The new feels distinctly different from the old, and in a short time, you accept the new, beneficial support.

How do I care for my new bed after I get it home?

Here are some guidelines for good mattress maintenance:

✦ Don't remove the tag. No, it's not illegal to remove it—just silly. You may need the information should you have a warranty claim.

- Follow your dealer's recommendations about turning the mattress. Some do not need to be turned, but most do, and you will void the warranty if you fail to turn it. (See diagram.) During the first 4 months, I recommend turning the mattress end-to-end and upside down every 2 weeks. Then, turn your mattress over and end-to-end every few months to equalize normal wear and tear.

- Turn the foundation end-to-end occasionally.

- Air out your mattress occasionally.

- Avoid bending the corners when putting on fitted sheets.

- Don't use dry-cleaning chemicals to remove spots or stains. The chemicals may harm the fabric or underlying materials. Use mild soap and cold water if you're really determined to try a clean-up. Apply it lightly; do not soak.

- Your bed is not a trampoline. Don't let kids jump on it; they could damage the interior construction, to say nothing of damaging themselves.

Now, I'll wrap up this chapter with some information about two favorite aspects of my work: open-cell foam (E-Foam) and adjustable beds.

How to Float on a Supportive Cloud

Please take note of E-Foam™, the Ergonomic Miracle. I think you'll be hearing much more about it. Some people call it Swedish foam, because it was originally incorporated into mattresses at Swedish hospitals. Hospital trials showed that it enhanced deep sleep, with 98 percent of the subjects reporting that their buttocks, loins, small of the back, and shoulders felt better on mattresses enhanced with the foam.[6]

E-Foam—also called memory foam—is an open-cell, porous, viscous material that "reads" your body's temperature and weight, and "gives" just the right amount to make you comfortable. The material conforms to your body, but always returns to its original shape. Some people can settle in almost instantly; for others, it takes from 5 to 10 minutes at the most for the most satisfying impression to be completed.

Open-cell foam offers pain-free, pressure-free sleep. You'll literally feel like you're floating on a cloud. The first NASA astronauts used this special material to lessen the impact of lift-offs and landings. Many U.S. medical professionals, such as doctors, chiropractors, and physical therapists, are now recommending this wonderful foam to alleviate back pain, arthritis pain, postsurgical pain, and many other problems. It is being used in hospital intensive care units, nursing homes, and, of course, in the homes of people who want extraordinary comfort and support.

When my daughter, Jennifer, was just out of college and beginning to work, she slept on a futon. She complained that her back was really hurting her, but she didn't have the money to buy a new bed. So I sent her an E-Foam topper, and it worked perfectly to clear up her pain.

"The electric bed is very comfortable with good back support and easy to use. We especially enjoy the fact that it does not look like a hospital bed. We commend your efforts to fill a definite need for a quality electric bed for those individuals who are not 'ill' per se but have a necessity for certain bedtime positions while trying to carry on a 'normal' lifestyle."
—Mr. and Mrs. James Toomer
Chesterfield, N.H.

You can buy pillows, mattress toppers, and mattresses made of E-Foam. If your current bed sags or really needs to be replaced, a mattress topper won't help it; it will just make the situation worse. But if your bed gives good support and you want to add some comfort while maintaining the support, an open-cell foam topper provides a wonderful solution. Standard sheets and pillow cases fit foam toppers and pillows just fine. E-Foam is also being used in the seats and arms of office chairs for a feeling of support and relaxation.

Adjustable Beds: Truly the Best

I believe the ideal bed exists in today's market. My husband and I have one ourselves: an adjustable bed with dual massage controls and a mattress that incorporates lots of E-Foam. We also have E-Foam pillows. With all this comfort, being in bed is pure heaven! After a hard day at work or when I don't feel well, there's nothing like climbing into bed, moving the position until it's just right, and breathing a deep sigh of relief. And all this before I even close my eyes to sleep!

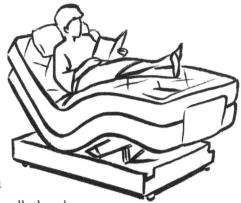

Adjustable beds have changed. They're not "hospital beds." They are beautifully designed furniture that add style and comfort to your bedroom. Some have a massage system that relieves tired, sore muscles and reduces tension. The controls are easy to hold, and the motors are quiet.

A Final Note

When you buy a new mattress set, you really are getting a great value compared to other items you purchase as a general consumer. When selected properly, as I've talked about in this chapter, your new bed will last years and years and give you a great deal of rest and comfort. The problem is that mattress manufacturers and many retailers have "lost their way" when they promote and merchandise mattresses. They often compete on price, price, price—but by now you know you need to buy based on benefits, benefits, benefits.

Remember, you probably spend more time in your bed than on any other piece of furniture. Make sure it supports your spine and gives you the best night's rest possible. You should look forward to going to sleep on it—and to waking up feeling refreshed and relaxed.

SUMMARY

I hope you now feel armed with enough information to start shopping for the new bed that will add hours of peace and comfort to your life. Here's a quick review:

✦ Test as many different mattresses as you need to until you find one with the right support and "feel." Wear loose, comfortable clothes and shoes that you can remove easily.

✦ Lie on your back and sides and as many other positions as you think you sleep in.

✦ Don't necessarily believe a manufacturer's label of "Firm" or "Plush." Try it for yourself, and put your own label of approval on the mattress that feels right to you.

✦ Buy the best bed you can afford. You'll always be able to find a bargain mattress, but it may be far from a bargain when it comes to pain-free, restful sleep.

Next, I'll cover some important information on arthritis, a pervasive, troublesome problem for millions of people.

CHAPTER 7

The Many Forms of Arthritis
How to Treat the Pain

"I joined the board of the Arthritis Foundation to help as many people as I can with what I've learned over the years about pain relief and how to make life easier. And in turn, the foundation has some excellent information and research to share, so I want to relay some of that to you here."

JoAnne

HIGHLIGHTS OF THIS CHAPTER

✦ Risk factors

✦ Fibromyalgia and other forms of arthritis

✦ Potential for a "cure"

✦ The mind-body connection

✦ Exercise and diet

✦ Alternative treatments

✦ Aids for pain relief

✦ List of information and support groups

S ome might consider it an epidemic. Arthritis currently affects more Americans than any other major disease except hypertension. More than 40 million Americans suffer from some form of arthritis—you won't believe how many disguises this disease has. The terms arthritis and rheumatism refer to mostly chronic conditions involving joint pain and inflamed, stiff muscles. Medically, these are defined as connective tissue diseases and rheumatic diseases. Many people suffer silently; many don't even know that the persistent ache or pain they have in a hand or joint can be labeled "arthritis."

Defining Arthritis

The two types of arthritis you hear about most often are osteoarthritis and rheumatoid arthritis.

Rheumatoid arthritis (RA) is an autoimmune disease in which the lining of the joints becomes inflamed. (Autoimmune means that the immune system malfunctions and the body essentially attacks itself.) Symptoms include stiffness, swelling, and pain, often around the small joints of the hands, wrists, elbows, shoulders, feet, and knees. There may also be evidence of systemic inflammation, such as fatigue, low-grade fever, weight loss, and anemia.

The cause of RA remains a mystery, although onset is frequently associated with physical or emotional stress. Rheumatoid arthritis can begin in childhood. Among adults, three times more women than men suffer from RA. Overall, it affects a small percentage (1 to 2 percent) of the population.[1] Treatment usually includes proper resting of the affected joints and medicine to control the inflammation and prevent joint destruction. More than two-thirds of those diagnosed with the disease go into remission within 2 years.

Osteoarthritis (OA), on the other hand, is not related to inflammation or immune system problems. The most common form of arthritis, it involves chemical and structural changes in cartilage, hardening of the bone, and formation of small bone spurs around the joints. By age 40, about 90 percent of the population show X-ray evidence of osteoarthritis in the weight-bearing joints, although symptoms usually do not begin until later in life.[2] Typically, OA affects joints such as the knees, hips, neck, lower back, and small joints of the hands. The breakdown of cartilage that comes with age leads the list of possible causes; obesity and joint trauma often precede the onset as well. Treatment includes simple analgesics such as acetaminophen or aspirin, and if those don't work, use of other nonsteroidal anti-inflammatory drugs or injections of corticosteroids to relieve the pain.

Is arthritis inherited? Well, your genetic makeup can influence your tendency to develop arthritis, but other factors also come into play. For example, you may be genetically susceptible to arthritis, but it might not show up unless you get an infection or your immune system malfunctions in some other way.

Obesity presents a major risk factor. According to the Centers for Disease Control and Prevention, obesity raises the risk of all types of arthritis (especially OA) by about 30 percent in both men and women. Your knees and hips, the primary weight-bearing joints of the body, can handle up to 2.5 to 10 times your weight.[3] So if you weigh 200 pounds, you may be putting up to a ton of pressure on your joints as you walk, run, or use them in daily life. Give your body a break. If you weigh too much, lose it!

Other Forms of Arthritis

Now, I don't want to alarm you or make you think you have some form of arthritis when you really don't, but I have a list of about 100 diagnoses that are associated with arthritis. The list includes diseases that you probably have heard of but may not know technically signify a form of arthritis, such as

- ✦ Carpal tunnel syndrome
- ✦ Crohn's disease
- ✦ Fibromyalgia
- ✦ Gout
- ✦ Lupus

- ✦ Lyme disease
- ✦ Myasthenia gravis
- ✦ Osteoporosis

Of course, there are other diseases or syndromes linked to arthritis that are rare and affect a small percentage of the population. Nevertheless, if you're one of those who knows you suffer from an arthritic condition, you welcome any information or remedies that will give you relief. My mission is to bring that information and those remedies to you in this book and through the products in my stores.

Many people live with some aspect of arthritis, knowingly or unknowingly. They enjoy normal lives, with an upbeat focus. If you have a "Woe is me" attitude about your health, it not only has a negative effect on the rest of your life and the lives of those around you, but it also prevents you from learning what you can do to conquer that pain or illness. So my job is to encourage you to learn how to take better care of yourself and improve your quality of life.

A Note on Fibromyalgia Syndrome

An estimated 7 to 10 million Americans, the majority of them women, suffer from the form of arthritis known as fibromyalgia syndrome (FMS), a term that means pain in the muscles, ligaments, and tendons—the fibrous tissues of our bodies. This pain can be very widespread and the fatigue that accompanies it can remain constant and overwhelming. Other symptoms of FMS include chronic headaches; stiffness throughout the body; cognitive difficulties with short-term memory; difficulty speaking or writing; problems with balance, vision, and digestion; allergic-like reactions; and hypersensitivity to weather patterns, light, noise, and pollutants.

The exact causes of FMS still pose a mystery, but the condition may occur after a viral infection, after unaccustomed and excessive physical activity, or during times of great emotional stress. Doctors diagnose the disease with criteria such as pain and tenderness in 11 of 18 specific trigger points on the body. But diagnosis also comes from excluding other causes. This is because tests on the symptoms often confuse the issue by coming up with normal results.

One of the most common symptoms of FMS shows up as sleep disturbances, or nonrestorative sleep. This might include sleep apnea, restless leg syndrome, or teeth gnashing. Sometimes drugs help this condition, but as a first line of attack, I would recommend improving your eating, exercise, and relaxation routines plus having a good mattress to send you off to a restful night's sleep. See chapter 1 for information on eating right, chapters 1 and 3 for help on exercise, chapter 5 on getting a good night's sleep, and chapter 6 for the latest in mattress technology.

Although there is no sure-fire cure for fibromyalgia, people who suffer from this disease can learn to live with it, manage it, and treat it. The symptoms may come and go, sometimes acting unruly, sometimes more under control. In *The Fibromyalgia Handbook*,[4] rheumatologist Harris H. McIlwain, M.D., describes his seven-step treatment program, which includes combinations of medicine, exercise, stress management, sound nutrition, and alternative therapies.

A Fibromyalgia Case Study

A young friend of mine, 34-year-old Jessica Mitchell, was diagnosed with fibromyalgia after experiencing severe muscle and joint pain for nearly 3 years. She had always been athletic, had worked out in step aerobics classes, and had played baseball and other sports. Her two young daughters and her volunteer work keep her hopping. I share her poignant story with you because her courage and determination inspire me. Let me quote from her letters written before the diagnosis:

> *I noticed my knees beginning to hurt when I did step aerobics . . . by February 1995, the pain became so bad I had to stop. I tried just walking and could not do that without pain. I have also noticed diminished strength in my arms. I have always helped my husband with a lot of the heavy lifting that's needed around the house, but it has become obvious*

that my lifting is hardly effective anymore. I cut back on all lifting or strenuous pushing and this seemed to help after about 4 weeks. However, when I tried to start up again gently, I noticed the pain beginning to increase, so I stopped doing things again.

On June 15, I was taking a plate out of a cabinet and experienced a terrible pain in my left elbow that made me drop the plate. I took some ibuprofen and the pain subsided some by that night. I had done nothing to overwork it or cause it any distress, yet this happened.

Beyond my joints and muscles, other things have me concerned. Earlier this year I started noticing a lot of my hair coming out in my hands when I washed it and on the floor when I dried it. In March and April my periods got super heavy, then became very short and light.... My face has been breaking out a lot more than usual, and I've also gained some weight. But a thyroid and hormone check showed these factors to be normal.

I know that stress can increase pain levels, and I have certainly had my share. Several people close to me died within a month.... I was president of my daughter's preschool, reading once a week at the elementary school and responsible for a class party and a fundraiser ... keeping three chiropractic appointments a week, attending church, and maintaining a household.

I've been taking it easy for 2 or 3 months now, minimal exertion and low stress, but these aches and pain continue. As a competitive athlete, I know what it is to have sore muscles after the first spring practice or tournament; this is not that. I've always been able to bounce back from things, but now it seems that once an area starts hurting, it doesn't stop, and the smallest bit of exertion aggravates it. I take as little medication as possible, try to resolve things naturally, and I eat well. I'm trying not to be overly nervous or preoccupied with this, but I am aware that something's going on and want to determine what it is.

In September 1997, a rheumatologist confirmed that Jessica has fibromyalgia, and this is how she's been since then:

In a way, some aspects of this illness are more annoying than painful. I couldn't have typed this letter 3 weeks ago because the tingling in my arms was so bad, I couldn't sit at the computer long enough to concentrate. I'm so glad the tingling and numbness have gone away, at least for now. Unfortunately, some pain, mild or intense, is always in my body.

I'm losing my hair again, too; however, I'm doing a good job of not letting it bother me. I think it's just my body's delayed response to the extreme stress I went through 6 months ago. You know the saying, "Don't wish for something too hard—you might get it." Well, I've always wished my hair weren't so thick, and now it's not!

I have reduced some of the stress in my life, I'm back to stepping more frequently, and my bedtime is now 10 p.m. I can get up on time in the mornings, do some stretches in bed, then get my children ready for school. I'm moderately active at church again. Occasionally, I take some ibuprofen for headaches. My new adjustable bed and the gel packs I warm in the microwave are doing wonders for my aches and pains.

As you can tell, this puzzling disease has many ups and downs. Jessica's attitude is remarkably upbeat, given what she's been through. Her case is not unusual, but I predict her outlook and faith will help her live her life fully as she copes with fibromyalgia.

The Arthritis *Cure*?

The best-selling book, *The Arthritis Cure*, by Dr. Jason Theodosakis, Brenda Adderly, and Barry Fox,[5] touts a program they claim can halt and even reverse the impact of osteoarthritis. It includes many of the ideas for health that I present in this book, and it highlights the use of two nutrients, glucosamine and chondroitin sulfates. The body manufactures these substances in small amounts. When taken as supplements, glucosamine and chondroitin have been used very successfully in other countries to reduce dramatically the pain of arthritis.

Even though the popularity of these nutrients is increasing here in the United States, many traditionally trained doctors discount the value of glucosamine and chondroitin. Yet Theodosakis and other prominent M.D.s[6] all cite research that shows promising results in patients who have pain from osteoarthritis.

Glucosamine and chondroitin ostensibly work to stop the breakdown of cartilage and to stimulate production of key elements of cartilage, thus enhancing repair and improving joint function. Theodosakis does not assert that this cures arthritis, but you might want to consider using these nutritional supplements as one approach to feeling better.

Living with Arthritis

While, at this point, there is no known cure for arthritis, no surefire remedy that magically and permanently takes away that nagging pain, many avenues have opened up. Research continues on several fronts, and there are ways to attack the pain and improve the quality of life for people who suffer from arthritis and its related syndromes. Of course, pharmaceutical companies are testing new drugs all the time, and informal support groups have sprung up all over the country. At the end of this chapter, you'll find a resource list of organizations providing information on arthritis and fibromyalgia. Now I want to talk with you about the numerous little things you can do for yourself (or a family member who has arthritis) that don't cost a lot of money and do enhance health.

"During an interview with JoAnne, I happened to mention that I have fibromyalgia. She suggested this high-tech, space age, memory foam mattress topper as something that might help. I gave it a serious personal test. For more than one month, I spent four nights sleeping with it on my bed in the city, and three nights without it in the country. Now I sleep much better in the city than I ever did in the country, and my symptoms have been relieved considerably."

—*Bob Madigan*
WTOP Newsradio
Washington, D.C.

Sleep on Open-Cell Foam, Not Air or Water

I've seen ads for ways to "sleep on air" by using a mattress with an air cushion, or ads for water beds that supposedly support your body. As you know if you read chapter 6, I don't agree with these at all. Yes, your body needs support, but it needs more than air or water. I believe you need the type of ergonomic, open-cell foam (E-Foam) that has been proven to enhance sleep and reduce pain (see chapter 6). It's sensitive to your body's weight and temperature, so the instant you lie down on it, it molds to your own body's curves, giving you support exactly where you need it while also providing enough flexibility for maximum comfort. A stiff mattress will just make you more uncomfortable, especially if you have the pain of fibromyalgia or arthritis.

Use Your Mind-Body Connection

Scientific research now documents that the way you think and feel definitely influences the way your body acts, physically and chemically. Every day, we learn something new about the brain and how it works. The pain you feel in your body is very real to you, even though at the moment there may be no physical evidence or manifestation of it. So don't let anyone dismiss you by saying, "It's all in your head." It may be all in your head, but that's just as important to you as if it's all in your body.

By using your mind consciously, you can cause chemical changes in your body that will minimize pain and maximize relaxation. Consider these techniques:

✦ *Meditation.* You don't have to have formal training or spend several years in India to make this work for you. Just pick a time of day to sit quietly, breathe deeply, and set aside your normal worries and activities. Focus either on your breath or on a pleasant thought or scene, such as your favorite beach or vacation setting, or soften your focus to nothing in particular. Let thoughts come and go and don't pay attention to what they mean. People have hundreds of different ways to meditate; different modes work for different people, so just find something that works for you. You might want to read a book on meditating or go to a class or group. I recommend that you start by carving out those few minutes each day to sit by yourself and enjoy doing nothing. It really makes a difference!

✦ *Deep breathing.* Dr. Herbert Benson was one of the first to document the physiological value of the "relaxation response." When you breathe slowly and deeply, using your abdominal muscles to bring air through your diaphragm instead of only through your chest, you trigger a series of physiological reactions that calm the body. These include a decrease in the pulse rate, blood pressure, respiration rate, oxygen consumption, and overall metabolism, all of which are beneficial for stress reduction and, ultimately, pain relief.

✦ *Yoga.* This ancient practice gently exercises your body and your mind. When you focus on deep breathing and coordinate it with body stretches and movements, you can relax and simultaneously relieve pain.

✦ *Laughter!* Dr. Norman Cousins was an early proponent of "laughter is the best medicine." In *Anatomy of An Illness,*[7] he discovered that "10 minutes of genuine belly laughter had an anesthetic effect and would give me at least 2 hours of pain-free sleep." Laughing also causes positive physiological changes and is guaranteed to make you forget about your pain for awhile. Watch a funny movie, spend some time with young children, or find someone who makes bad puns, and you'll change your view of life by laughing at it.

Relax!

In addition to the above paths that lead to relaxation, you can take more active steps to remove your focus from pain.

✦ *Get a massage.* Ask a family member or friend to put some soothing hands on you, or schedule a professional massage session. Massage increases the circulation of blood to sore and tender areas, relaxes muscles in spasm, and eases tension. You can even massage yourself with the intention of relieving pain and relaxing. There are many battery-powered and electric massagers on the market that bring relief to every part of the body, especially those you can't reach with your hands.

✦ *Take a bath.* There's nothing like a warm bath to soothe aches and pains. Yes, even for men, too! Find a hot tub, climb into a whirlpool, or just step into your bathtub and soak for a few peaceful minutes, turning your mind to something that makes you happy.

✦ *Listen to music.* Pick whatever turns you on. For some people, it's rock music that energizes them; for others, it's classical music that energizes, inspires, or brings peace.

Exercise!

It used to be that people with arthritis were advised to refrain from vigorous exercise and do only gentle range-of-motion movements in order to "save their joints" from further destruction. Times have changed. Now the experts encourage all three major types of exercise: aerobic, strengthening, and range of motion. According to Dr. Theodosakis, exercise fights the debilitating effects of osteoarthritis in two major ways:[8]

1. It encourages the flow of synovial fluid into and out of the cartilage. This is the essential fluid that lubricates and nourishes the cartilage, keeping it moist and healthy.

2. It strengthens supporting structures (muscles, tendons, ligaments) and increases the range of motion, shock absorption, and flexibility of the joints. The stronger these supporting structures are, the less pressure the joints must bear as you move.

As long as you protect your joints a bit, you can do almost any type of exercise and stretching that feels good. This will result in a healthier body, less pain, and improved immune function. Just remember that if you have a temporary inflammation, don't work that joint or part of the body. Wait until the soreness ebbs, then slowly start exercising it again. The latest government exercise guidelines declare that you can spread out your aerobic activity over the course of the day, as long as you get at least 30 minutes of moderate activity each day. That's good news for anyone who may be trying to loosen up stiff, achy joints. Do a little bit at a time and keep yourself pain free over a period of many hours.

Eat a Healthy Diet

You just can't escape from this advice, can you? Some people say that avoiding certain foods, such as those in the nightshade family (potatoes, tomatoes, eggplant, and bell peppers), helps arthritis. Although there doesn't seem to be any solid scientific evidence for this, maybe it's true for you. Overall, the best way to eat is to follow these guidelines:

✦ *Concentrate on low- or no-fat foods.* Work especially diligently to eliminate saturated fat from your diet.

✦ *Pack in those fruits and veggies.* The more, the better. They have fiber, vitamins, minerals, and all sorts of health-enhancing, disease-preventing nutrients. Foods that contain antioxidants (such as vitamins A, C, E, and selenium) may be especially desirable because these nutrients help fight the free radical molecules that are thought to attack and destroy the tissue in joints.

✦ *Get enough Omega-3 essential fatty acids.* These help reduce inflammation. Fish such as salmon and sardines are high in Omega-3s; so is flaxseed and flaxseed oil.

✦ *Drink lots of water.* Go for 6 to 8 glasses a day. Keep a glass on your desk if you work there during the day, or carry a bottle with you so you'll be able to sip it slowly and continuously.

✦ *Try to eat more fiber.* You'll find it in whole grain breads, cereals, and pastas, and in legumes (beans, dried peas). Nutritionists recommend that you consume 25–35 grams of fiber each day; most people average only about 11 grams.

- *Cut down on sugar.* Some experts claim sugar is as damaging to health and immunity as fat. Sugar appears in just about every processed food you buy, from peanut butter and ketchup to salad dressing and even canned vegetables.

Of course, the bonus of eating this way is either weight loss (if you're overweight) or weight maintenance. Keeping those extra pounds off is crucial to living with arthritis and even to preventing it, because your joints will have less pressure on them.

Use Alternative Therapies

I know that when I'm in pain, I'll do almost anything to get relief. I'm positive many arthritis sufferers confront the same situation and look beyond drugs for other ways to relieve pain or even cure the disease. Alternative medicine is becoming more and more common and not just for arthritis patients. More than a third of Americans have used some form of alternative medicine or treatment—everything from herbs and vitamins to chiropractic and acupuncture.

It's fine to keep an open mind and experiment, but I also recommend that you proceed with caution and make sure you can retreat if necessary. Look for new products, ideas, and treatments that have a good initial track record and that don't require a huge monetary investment. Talk with people who have used them, talk with your doctor if you wish, and then make up your own mind.

With that said, let me list several treatments or "modalities" that people tell me they find extremely helpful in their battle with arthritis. For the people who use these successfully, they are not even considered to be alternative medicine.

- *Meditation.* As I've suggested, this is an excellent way to calm the mind and the body.
- *Acupuncture.* This centuries-old, minimally invasive technique from the Orient has proven very effective in relieving pain. Acupuncture restores

balance to the various physical and energetic parts of the body. The Chinese believe that when your energy is out of balance, illness results.

✦ *Chiropractic.* Some medical doctors strongly oppose chiropractic and claim it potentially could harm people with osteoporosis and other forms of arthritis that affect the spine. If you have doubts, talk to both your medical doctor and a doctor of chiropractic before you act.

✦ *Biofeedback.* This method offers a clear demonstration of how the mind affects the body. During biofeedback, electronic sensors measure your body's automatic functions like muscle tension, pulse rate, and skin temperature. When you see the data from these measurements and practice relaxing, you can then consciously affect these functions to regulate your blood pressure, heart rate, muscle tension, and skin temperature.

The Arthritis Foundation endorses the above treatments as "complementary," meaning that several reliable scientific studies back them up, and they often are used in conjunction with standard medical treatment. The Foundation also cautions **against** the following treatments because they are unproven and potentially harmful:

✦ *Black Pearl.* Contains undisclosed ingredients that may be harmful.

✦ *Snake or bee venom.* May precipitate a severe allergic reaction.

✦ *DMSO (Dimethyl Sulfoxide).* Very controversial, with conflicting results. May cause severe side effects.

✦ *Commercial lubricants.* WD-40® is one example. May ease pain in some people when applied topically, but could cause skin rashes and burns. Do not take orally.

Aids for Pain Relief

You can buy many products to ease your pain. They range from a small ball you hold in your palm to major pieces of furniture such as adjustable beds. Here are just a few suggestions:

- ✦ *Exercise Ball.* Heat this small, pliable ball in the microwave for a few seconds, then work it around your palm and fingers for greater flexibility and soothing warmth.

- ✦ *Gel Wraps.* These are gel packs shaped to the various parts of your body: your neck, lower back, wrist, knee, etc. You can heat them for a minute in the microwave or keep them cold in the freezer. Wrap them around the painful area for 20 minutes, use their handy Velcro™ fasteners, and go about your daily life. Of course, be careful not to overheat the gel packs, and do not use them cold if you have circulation problems or decreased sensation.

- ✦ *Open-cell foam, or E-Foam™.* It is weight- and temperature-sensitive, and molds to the curves in your body, giving pain-free support. It is built into pillows, desk chairs, and mattress toppers (pads), and even mattresses. Trust me; you'll love it.

- ✦ *The Embracer Mattress by Spine-Align.* It's made with a touch of silk and wool and features posture-zone foam for truly ergonomic body support. I designed this myself.

> *"I've noticed a vast improvement in my circulatory and arthritic ailments since I've utilized the specialized [adjustable] bed not only at night, but for mid-day rests."*
>
> —*Frances F. DiBitetto*
> *Waldorf, Md.*

- ✦ *Adjustable beds.* The ultimate in support, these beds raise your back and knees to any position that's comfortable for you. They promote healthy circulation,

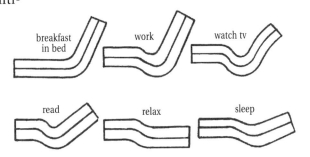

breakfast in bed   work   watch tv

read   relax   sleep

ease back pain, and offer great relief. Change the position for reading, watching TV, eating, or sleeping. I know many people with arthritis who adore their adjustable beds and don't know how they ever lived without them. Since the body is capable of nearly infinite positions and levels of discomfort, why not match that with a bed capable of nearly infinite positions and levels of comfort?

SUMMARY

The most common form of arthritis, osteoarthritis, affects some 40 million Americans. Other forms of arthritis include rheumatoid arthritis, fibromyalgia, gout, lupus, and lyme disease. Arthritis can cause extensive pain and affect its victims' quality of life.

Treatments vary widely and include aspirin, acetaminophen or other nonsteroidal anti-inflammatory drugs, and sometimes corticosteroids. Nondrug remedies range from supplements such as glucosamine and chondroitin to mind-body techniques and alternative therapies such as acupuncture and biofeedback. Getting proper exercise and eating well bring clear-cut benefits to managing arthritis. Finally, an open-cell foam mattress topper or an adjustable bed adds major ongoing comfort for anyone in pain.

Next, a short discussion of another category of pain, carpal tunnel syndrome and repetitive motion injuries.

Health Information and Support Groups

This list is from the *Johns Hopkins White Paper* on arthritis.[9]

**American Academy of
  Orthopaedic Surgeons**
6300 N. River Road
Rosemont, IL 60018-4262
800-346-2267
www.aaos.org

Arthritis Foundation
1330 W. Peachtree St.
Atlanta, GA 30309
800-283-7800
www.arthritis.org

**Fibromyalgia Alliance
  of America**
P.O. Box 21990
Columbus, OH 43221-0990
1-888-717-6711

Lupus Foundation of America
1300 Piccard Dr., Suite 200
Rockville, MD 20850-4303
800-558-0121
www.lupus.org/lupus

**National Institute of Arthritis
  & Musculoskeletal
  & Skin Diseases
  Information Clearinghouse**
National Institutes of Health
One AMS Circle
Bethesda, MD 20892-3675
301-495-4484
www.nih.gov/niams

**National Institute on Aging
  Information Center**
P.O. Box 8057
Gaithersburg, MD 20898-8057
800-222-2225
www.nih.gov/nia

CHAPTER 8

Carpal Tunnel Syndrome and Repetitive Motion Injuries

What You Can Do About Them

"The good news is that these problems can be treated successfully, especially if diagnosed early, and they can be prevented when you take care of yourself. For example, I recommend a wrist pad for your computer keyboard. Or attach a protective armrest to your chair or desk."

JoAnne

HIGHLIGHTS OF THIS CHAPTER

✦ Symptoms of carpal tunnel syndrome

✦ Other repetitive stress injuries

✦ Students and computer use

✦ Getting the right diagnosis

✦ Nonsurgical treatments

✦ Ergonomic factors

✦ Guidelines for wrist health

W e seem to hear a lot these days about carpal tunnel syndrome (CTS), a problem that many people have experienced as they use their wrists for the same movements hour after hour, day after day. CTS occurs when a nerve that supplies power and feeling to the hand becomes compressed in the narrow "tunnel," the passageway through the wrist.

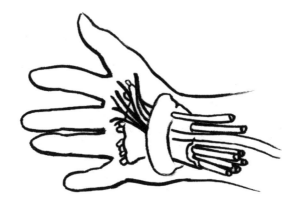

Numbness in the thumb and first two fingers often signals the beginning of CTS. Additional symptoms include tingling, more numbness, and severe pain. Sometimes, the symptoms are so severe that you can't sleep at night. The syndrome may appear after an injury such as a fall or fracture. Or it can result from repetitive movements like typing, using a vibrating tool, working on an assembly line, or using a scanner at the supermarket. In other cases, edema, or fluid retention, may cause swelling of the tissue or even of the nerve in the carpal tunnel. This occurs most often in pregnancy; the symptoms subside after delivery.

Carpal tunnel syndrome actually fits into a larger class of problems called repetitive motion injuries, repetitive stress or strain injuries, or cumulative trauma disorders. The Bureau of Labor Statistics (BLS) reports that cases of such repetitive stress injuries now account for 65 percent of all occupational illnesses, with CTS comprising nearly half of these.[1] All these complaints are difficult to diagnose accurately. Many people have surgery for CTS, but it often doesn't clear up their pain.

Great controversy surrounds repetitive motion injuries and CTS, not only from a medical point of view, but also from the economic implications. According to one estimate, repetitive motion complaints cost American industry at least $20 billion a year in worker's compensation costs.[2] Some experts say these complaints come from our increasing use of high technology and automation and from the focus on maximum productivity in the workplace. Many people sit at computer keyboards all day long, probably without paying much attention to posture or to getting up and stretching every once in a while.

In fact, with kids starting to use computers at younger and younger ages, the risk of repetitive motion complaints is rising. Reports of repetitive stress injuries (RSI) among high school and college students are increasing.[3] Some schools have started education and prevention campaigns; others are providing note-takers and voice-recognition software, which allows students with RSI to dictate their work.

Getting the Right Diagnosis

Numbness, tingling, and pain that many patients initially attribute to carpal tunnel syndrome may not be that at all. These are also symptoms of the more general category of repetitive stress injuries. One estimate claims that the nerve test for CTS inaccurately identifies about 15 percent of patients.[4] In other words, results of the test could show you have CTS when in fact you do not.

On the other hand, when CTS is ruled out, many doctors are unable to attribute their patients' neck, shoulder, arm, or hand pain to a specific physiological explanation. A problem called Thoracic Outlet Syndrome also causes tingling, weakness, numbness, and pain in the arms and hands due to the pinching or restriction of nerves or arteries between the spinal column and the ribs. Make sure you don't get treatment or surgery for a carpal tunnel problem when it's really something else.

So when you group carpal tunnel problems with other repetitive stress injuries, you come up with lots of pain, difficulties in diagnosis, and high cost of treatment. Many people can avoid surgery with exercises, physical therapy, acupuncture, or massage techniques. Other treatments include splinting, anti-inflammatory medication, and adjusting the work station and work habits. Vitamin B_6, at 100 milligrams per day, has helped in some cases. Experts say it's important to have minimal muscle tension when you type or perform similar repetitive motions. Patients can learn how to relax their muscles using biofeedback techniques. In some cases of repetitive stress injuries, there are nonoccupational risk factors to address such as diabetes, obesity, smoking, or a thyroid condition.

Remember ergonomics, the science of fitting the environment to you rather than making you conform to the environment? Ergonomics experts contend that sitting up straight at a computer keyboard works the muscles harder than most people realize. Just keeping your fingers prepared for typing without flopping them on the keyboard requires contraction of the arm and shoulder muscles, which impedes blood flow. Poor posture, as you know, can cause strain in the neck, shoulder, back, and even leg muscles.

Guidelines for Wrist Health

Well, if I haven't frightened you enough, I want to talk about how to take care of yourself and avoid repetitive stress injuries and carpal tunnel syndrome. Here are some tips:

- ✦ "Warm up" your wrists before any stressful activity. Stretch your hands and wrists in different positions and hold them gently for a few seconds. Separate the fingers as widely as you can and hold for a few seconds.
- ✦ Keep your whole body in good shape, paying attention to circulation, posture, and breathing.
- ✦ Use the entire hand (or both of them) and all the fingers to pick things up and grasp objects if possible. Using only your thumb and index finger can put stress on your wrist. Use tools and equipment that correctly fit your hand size.

- Hold your wrists in a neutral position when typing, not angled up or down from the keyboard. Try a wrist rest that fits against your keyboard, or arm extenders on your chair. (See diagram below.) Hold your computer mouse loosely and avoid typing too hard.

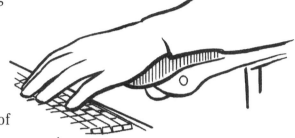

- Review the diagrams in chapter 4 for correct sitting posture, either at your desk or in front of your computer: your video screen is from about 18 up to 30 inches in front of you; your eyes are level with the top third of the screen; your back is straight; your knees are slightly tipped up with feet flat on the floor (or on a foot rest if you need it); your keyboard is at a height that leaves your arms and wrists horizontal.

- Give your hands, arms, and neck a break every now and then; do a different task, use different muscles, stand up and stretch. Check out Stretch Break™, a program you install on your computer that reminds you to stretch at preprogrammed intervals and displays the stretches on your screen. As you install this program, you select how long you want to wait between stretch sessions and how many stretches you want to do during each session. Each stretch lasts for 15 to 25 seconds, so you can break for a minute or two or for longer if you wish.

- When you carry or hold a baby (or some other object) in the "cradle" position, also hold something with the fingers of the lifting hand. For example, grip the edge of the blanket or a diaper wrap. According to the authors of *How to Raise Children Without Breaking Your Back*, this protects your wrist, because you can't close your fist all the way

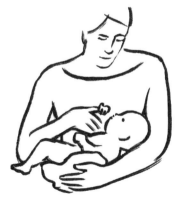

when you also grip something with your fingers.[5] Staying too long in a closed-wrist, flexed position can strain the delicate wrist muscles.

✦ The string game, Cat's Cradle, works as an excellent wrist conditioner!

✦ Finally, if you think you may have a carpal tunnel or other repetitive stress injury, do get professional help or evaluation. The earlier a problem is diagnosed, the better the chances are for recovery.

SUMMARY

Carpal tunnel syndrome and other repetitive stress injuries are becoming more prevalent as people work more with computers and other streamlined technology. Even young kids and older students who spend many hours in front of their computers are at risk.

Many nonsurgical options are available, including exercise, physical therapy, massage, and splinting. Adjusting the work station and work habits often helps greatly. With good posture, attention to wrist position, and other preventive measures, you can take good care of your wrists and arms to avoid the pain of repetitive stress injuries.

To wrap up my advice to you in this book, I want to touch on some important back-related topics that you might encounter every day: caring for kids, traveling, and managing stress.

CHAPTER 9

Back Care in Daily Life

Coping with Kids, Travel, and Stress

"Everyone needs back care. I've heard complaints about backaches from 8-year-olds, from teens, from mothers-to-be, from baby boomers, and from senior citizens. By paying attention to our bodies, it is definitely possible not only to relieve pain but also to prevent it in the first place."

JoAnne

HIGHLIGHTS OF THIS CHAPTER

✦ Back care during pregnancy

✦ When the baby arrives

✦ Packing for comfortable travel

✦ Avoiding back pain in cars and on planes

✦ What to do when you arrive

✦ The ultimate stress management tip

✦ Yoga for stress relief

Pregnancy and Your Back

Nine months may seem like a long time to wait for a baby to be born, but a woman's body needs to go through some major changes in order for the great event to take place. The usually stable joints of the pelvis start loosening up to allow easier passage for the baby at delivery. This change, along with the ever-expanding abdomen, throws the body off balance. A woman often unconsciously compensates for this by arching her neck and bringing her shoulders back. Her lower back can then become deeply curved, resulting in strained muscles and back pain.

The following advice comes from the popular book *What to Expect When You're Expecting*.[1] Not only is it helpful for pregnant women but it also provides good guidance for anyone who wants a healthy back!

✦ Try to keep weight gain within recommended limits. Excess pounds, even when you're not pregnant, always put a strain on the lower back.

✦ Wear shoes with good support. Say goodbye to high heels, maybe forever; they throw your spine out of alignment.

✦ Learn proper ways to lift, and don't pick up loads that are too heavy. Bend at the knees, not at the waist, and rely on your arm and leg muscles, not your back, when you lift.

✦ Alternate between your right and left sides when carrying things, or divide a heavy load into two and carry one package on each side.

✦ Try not to stand for long periods of time. If you must, keep one foot propped on a low stool to prevent low back strain (like the cowboys used to do as they stood at the bar in a saloon).

✦ Don't stretch your arms too far above your head (to put dishes away in a cupboard, for example). Instead, use a low, sturdy footstool. Reaching too far strains back muscles.

✦ Follow my chapter 4 suggestions for proper alignment when sitting. Avoid backless stools and benches. And, please, don't cross your legs when you sit. This not only impedes circulation, but it also can cause you to tilt your pelvis too far forward and contribute to a backache.

♦ Sleep on your left side (this aids circulation), with a pillow wedged between your legs to support your belly. When you get out of bed, swing both legs over the side of the bed and, at the same time, use your arms to lift your upper body. See chapter 5 for more suggestions on sleeping comfortably when you're pregnant.

> "We bought our adjustable bed about 2 years before I got pregnant, and boy, did it help during my pregnancy. It was a great aid in taking pressure off my back and getting a good night's sleep. Now I lift the top of the bed when I breast feed, then lower it so my little girl and I can take a nap."
> —Mindy Griffiths
> Vienna, Va.

♦ Do exercises to strengthen your abdominal muscles. In fact, keep all your muscles as well toned and exercised as you safely can.

When the Baby Arrives

With all the attention focused on your new bundle of joy, many parents don't have much time to take care of themselves or think it's not important, or both. Nothing could be further from the truth! It takes a healthy parent to raise a healthy child. This means it's no good to have a father whose back hurts so much that he snaps at his kid or a mother who tries to do so many things that her own stress makes her kids anxious. So if you are a parent, recruit family and friends, and even your children as they grow to understand, to help you stay mentally and physically healthy by getting good sleep and eating right.

We don't carry a lot of books, but I found *How to Raise Children Without Breaking Your Back* to be so outstanding that I now offer it in my stores.[2] The book includes everything from recovering from C-sections and retoning your muscles to proper positions for nursing, carrying, and changing the baby to ways to take care of yourself and heal physical injuries and mental stress. It has lots of exercises, diagrams, and lists of resources for further information. Fathers can benefit from it too. Here are a few pointers from this wonderful book.

+ *Feeding your baby.* During feeding times, parents tend to look down adoringly at their babies. This creates an incredible strain on the neck. To counteract it, shift the baby from side to side, remember to look up and around regularly, and use gentle exercises to stretch and tone your neck muscles. Support your back with a pillow if necessary.

+ *Changing diapers.* By the time your child turns 2, you will have changed approximately 4,000 diapers! You can see why it's important to have a changing table that is safe and feels comfortable. Setting the surface at waist height puts the table about right for most people. Too high a table makes it hard on the upper back, too low strains the lower and middle back. Beds are normally too low for changing; if you want to use the bed, climb up on it yourself and kneel or sit by the baby to give you correct leverage.

+ *Moving your baby.* Move your baby off the changing table and other surfaces slowly and carefully, paying attention not only to the baby's safety but also to your own body mechanics and the alignment of your spine. Twisting and lifting at the same time is the "worst possible combination of movements for your spine." Here is the wrong way to do it.

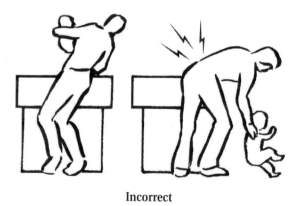

Incorrect

Instead, lift, take a breath, and then move your feet to begin your turn.

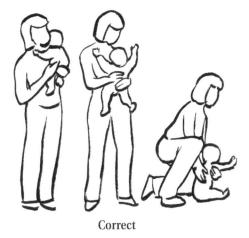

Correct

✦ *Picking up your baby.* Bending over to pick up or put your baby in a play-pen or low crib can be a backbreaker. Here is the safe way to do it.

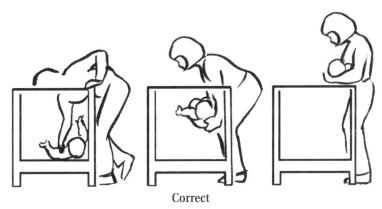

Correct

✦ *Maneuvering with car seats.* Putting babies and young children in and out of car seats places great strain on parents' backs. The safest way to do it keeps the child as close to your body as possible when you lift. One way to accomplish this would be to place the car seat in the center of the back seat and sit next to your child as you lift him onto your lap. Then slide over to the door, put both feet on the ground, and stand up, holding your child close. Another way would be to place the car seat next to the door so you can reach down and scoop her up, holding her close to your body. Then back out. Some car seats are built to swivel, which would make this action even easier.

There are many other ways to take loving care of your baby and protect your body at the same time. Much of the secret is common sense; the rest is some knowledge of body mechanics and some practice with basic exercises and stretches. Take action to prevent problems now, and you will be running around with your children—and their children—when you're "over the hill," whenever you consider that to be!

Now, here are some tips for another important area of life.

Travel and Your Back

I've discovered all sorts of ways to minimize the inconvenience and even pain that some people associate with travel. Now when I travel, I concentrate on having fun. Yet I know that leaving the comfort and safety of home produces instant stress for some folks, stress that tightens the back or tenses the neck. Keeping an irregular schedule, sleeping on unfamiliar beds, and not having access to your accustomed foods and exercise can all be unsettling. But there are lots of things you can do to take care of and even pamper yourself while you're on the road—things that will allow you to focus on the business or vacation at hand.

Packing

✦ Use a suitcase that rolls on its own wheels if possible. This will save your back from heavy lifting chores. As you pull it along, be sure to keep it close to your body, which promotes good body mechanics.

✦ Take comfortable clothes if you need to be in a car or on a bus, train, or plane for a few hours. Make sure you can stretch in them, and wear shoes that can carry you on a brief, brisk exercise walk when you take a break.

✦ Bring water and healthy snacks so you will be able to enjoy the trip and not worry about being thirsty or hungry. Pretzels, low-fat trail mix, a granola bar, fruit, and carrot and celery sticks hold up for many hours. I'm sure you can add your own favorite foods.

◆ Make room for a travel pillow. A travel pillow is worth more than its weight in gold—it's worth its space! There's nothing like having a pillow you're used to when you lay your head down on a bed that isn't your own.

◆ Consider bringing along an inflatable neck pillow to use for naps while you're on your way to your destination. Remember, I'm relentless when it comes to the absolute necessity of keeping your spine aligned. Believe me, you don't want to wake up from a nap with a crick in your neck or back.

> *"I want to thank you for all the help you gave me in fitting me with a back support device for my car. I was in a bad car accident and have had back problems for the last 3 years. The lower lumbar support device you suggested has helped me greatly."*
>
> —*James Bohuslaw*
> *Bohemia, N.Y.*

◆ Pack your jump rope or stretchable bands if you use them to exercise. How lightweight can you get? Some people take their exercise video or audiotapes. It's all a matter of being committed to the exercise that makes you feel good and keeps you energized and healthy.

◆ Consider bringing back rests, lumbar pillows, and footrests, which are all portable. For people who have back and neck pain, these are often indispensable parts of a trip; they make the difference between enjoyment and agony.

Pain-Free Car Travel

◆ Stretch as often as you can and definitely in the morning before you even get into the car. There are lots of good stretches for the spine (see Bob Anderson's excellent book *Stretching*).

◆ Take a break every hour or so. Get out of the car at a rest stop and walk around for a few minutes. Breathe deeply! Reach up in the air and down toward your toes.

◆ Keep the car at a cool temperature. When people are too warm, they become irritable, and the stress can go right into the back.

- Use a lumbar support, wedge, or car support that helps align your spine. Your car's seats are designed for looks, not comfort. It always amazes me to see how many people benefit from lumbar supports in their cars. That's often the first solution I suggest when I hear complaints about low back pain.

Airports and Planes

- Try this trick to avoid jet lag, based on the fact that body rhythms experience more trouble on eastward journeys than on westward ones. Before a long trip east, go to bed and get up an hour earlier each day for 3 days; before a long trip west, go to bed and get up an hour later each day for 3 days.

- Stretch as many parts of your body as you can while you wait for your plane or when you're between flights. Don't worry—people are looking at you in envy that you do these stretches to take care of yourself (or maybe nobody's looking anyway).

- Walk from one end of the terminal to the other, or maybe even outside when you have time and weather on your side.

- Stretch gently while seated, and get up once an hour to walk up and down the aisle during your flight. One of my friends goes to the front of the coach cabin and pretends to look out the porthole window in the door as she stretches her hamstrings; then she lifts up her lower legs to stretch her quads. You get the idea.

- Avoid things that interfere with good sleep on your journey. Avoid caffeine, alcohol, and heavy meals when you fly. Also, drink plenty of water and other fluids to counteract the dehydrating atmosphere on the plane.

When You Arrive

- Ask the hotel or whomever you're staying with for an extra pillow to put under your knees when you sleep. You may not need it once you get in bed, but it's easier to be prepared.

- Try to keep the hours of your new location if you're in a different time zone than your home zone. If you've flown through the night and arrived in the morning, have breakfast and try to stay awake all day. This will help your body adapt more quickly to the new time.

- Stretch, walk, or engage in heavier exercise to work the kinks of traveling from your body. This will also help you sleep better when the time comes.

- Get outside in the daylight for awhile. Light plays a key role in regulating your internal body rhythms, so use it to reset your biological clock.

- Have a professional massage, or ask a friend or family member to give you one. Even a 5-minute shoulder rub helps relax muscles and the mind.

Finally, I want to touch on stress management, that magical process that may seem so elusive. Once you sincerely make up your mind to take some stress out of your life, it doesn't have to be difficult. All the advice I've given you in this book (eating well, exercising, getting a good night's sleep, paying attention to your own needs) will help reduce stress. Now, here are some additional suggestions.

The Ultimate Stress Management Tip

A good friend of mine, Dr. Mort Orman of Baltimore, Md., has written an excellent book, *The 14-Day Stress Cure.* And even though he hates to give quick little tips to lessen stress, he agreed to write the "mother of all tips" for a recent issue of his newsletter. Actually, he says this piece of wisdom is not a tip at all, not a simple prescription you can mechanically follow to relieve any stressful situation. Rather, it is a starting point, a way to orient your thinking. Here it is:

Learn to appreciate the value of being wrong!

This doesn't sound like too much fun, does it? But if you take a closer look, as I did after I read Mort's newsletter, you will see that people are more often "wrong" than "right" and that everyone can learn from this. Mort teaches that people are biologically programmed to be wrong. For example, our eyes see only a fraction of the total light spectrum emitted by the sun; human ears hear a more limited range of sound than many other animals. Rather than being arrogant about this, people can appreciate it, and look for ways to compensate.

There are many other ways people persist in being wrong, according to Mort, such as thinking they know what others are truly thinking or feeling, what others are capable of achieving, or what people are really committed to in their lives. When they realize that they don't necessarily know the truth, it liberates them from the stress of anger-producing conversations and other negative situations. Mort affirms that appreciating the value of being wrong is nothing to be ashamed of; rather, it can be a profitable self-management tool that leads to openness and exhilaration.

> *I used to be terribly afraid of making mistakes, because I didn't want to be wrong. This caused a lot of stress in my life, especially in my business. But after reading Mort's wise words, I'm not so upset if I do make a mistake. I just look to see what I can learn from it and move on. Life is much less stressful this way.*

The Benefits of Yoga

Many people, both men and women, are turning to yoga these days for stress relief and muscle stretching and strengthening. Really, anyone can do the simpler yoga exercises—you don't have to be an Indian swami and tie yourself up into knots to get the benefits of yoga! And as I've said, one of the main benefits comes from concentrating on your breathing as you do the stretches and positions slowly and luxuriously, sending health-giving oxygen into all the nooks and crannies of your body.

In *Back Care Basics: A Doctor's Gentle Yoga Program for Back and Neck Pain Relief*,[5] Dr. Mary Pullig Schatz (no relation to me) rolls out a carefully planned, comprehensive program for healing the back. She emphasizes the importance of assessing your current state of flexibility and paying attention to the principles of body mechanics and proper alignment before attempting any of the yoga poses. In this well-illustrated book, Dr. Schatz assures you that using each pose to create inner quietness and peace will move you toward healing and rejuvenation.

Relaxation in a Bag

For some instant stress relief, listen to a relaxation audiotape such as the one in Shelly Greenberg's Relaxation in a Bag®. It contains a silk eye pillow and an audiotape that guides you into a 20-minute minivacation whenever you choose. You can lie down and rest the pillow over your eyes while listening to the soothing instructions on the tape. Or you can use the kit's adjustable travel band to secure the pillow when your head is in an upright position, such as in your car at a rest stop or on an airplane.

However you relax and manage the stress in your life, remember that you are important—to yourself and to the people who love you. So take good care of yourself!

SUMMARY

Awareness of good posture and care of the spine isn't limited to people with back pain. In daily life, there are hundreds of opportunities to care for yourself and prevent back pain. From pregnancy to child care to car and plane travel, you can easily monitor your movements to protect your back and neck. All it takes is awareness, determination, and a little practice. Yoga and conscious relaxation offer wonderful paths to self-care and healing.

Stress management also requires some awareness, determination, practice, and perhaps this basic wisdom from Dr. Mort Orman: Learn to appreciate the value of being wrong. This will open up the possibility of learning more about yourself and others.

My final words to you are "It's all going to work out." Mark Twain once said, "I have been through some terrible things in my life, some of which actually happened." Our minds can make up gruesome scenarios about what could happen to us, or our minds incorrectly perceive what is happening to us, but many of these fears do not reflect the truth. So just relax. Try to live in the present moment, appreciating what's good about your life and working to change what doesn't please you. Be kind to your body. Express your love to others. It's all going to work out.

JoAnne

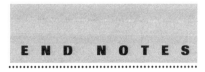

CHAPTER 1
The Good Health Triangle

1. Gabe Mirkin and Diana Rich, *Fat Free, Flavor Full* (New York: Little, Brown & Co., 1995). I found this book to be so valuable that I'm now offering it in all my stores.

2. The Boston-based Oldways Preservation and Exchange Trust, in consultation with researchers from Harvard and Cornell, has published two more pyramids. In the "Mediterranean Diet Pyramid," animal foods make up a much smaller proportion of the recommended daily food intake. And in the "Vegetarian Diet Pyramid," the emphasis is on plant foods: legumes, grains, fruits, and vegetables.

3. Evelyn Tribole and Elyse Resch, *Intuitive Eating: A Recovery Book for the Chronic Dieter* (New York: St. Martin's Press, 1995).

4. Studies quoted in Miriam E. Nelson, Ph.D., *Strong Women Stay Young* (New York: Bantam Books, 1998), 246.

5. Bob Anderson, *Stretching* (Bolinas, Calif.: Shelter Publications, 1980).

6. Morton C. Orman, M.D., *Dr. Orman's Guide to Better Sleep* (Baltimore, Md.: TRO Publications, 1995). Contact Dr. Mort Orman at <www.stresscure.com>.

7. We are grateful to the Better Sleep Council for assistance on this book. For more information, contact the Better Sleep Council, P.O. Box 19534, Alexandria, VA 22320-0534, or on the Web at <www.bettersleep.org>.

8. Andrew Weil, M.D., *Spontaneous Healing* (New York: Alfred A. Knopf, 1995), 212.

CHAPTER 2
Back and Neck Pain 101

1. Papageorgiou et al., quoted in *Bone Scan*, newsletter of Dr. Mark Smith, Vienna, Va., (April/May 1996).

2. Courtesy of Ergoworks Consulting, Gaithersburg, Md.

3. U.S. Public Health Service (USPHS) Agency for Health Care Policy and Research, *Understanding Acute Low Back Problems*. Obtain a copy by writing to the agency's Publications Clearinghouse, P.O. Box 8547, Silver Spring, MD 20907, or calling 1-800-358-9295.

4. Simeon Margolis, M.D., and John Kostuik, M.D., *The Johns Hopkins White Papers: Low Back Pain* (New York: Medletter Associates, Inc., 1997), 16.

5. Lewis G. Maharam, M.D., *A Healthy Back* (New York: Henry Holt & Co., 1996), 64.

6. Margolis and Kostuik, *Low Back Pain*, 8.

7. Ibid., 40.

CHAPTER 3

How to Get Your Back on Its Feet *and* Prevent Future Pain

1. Margolis and Kostuik, *Low Back Pain*, 17.

2. See USPHS Agency for Health Care Policy and Research, *Understanding Acute Low Back Problems*, loc. cit.

3. Adapted from Alex Pirie and Hollis Herman, *How to Raise Children without Breaking Your Back* (Somerville, Mass.: IBIS Publications, 1995), 49.

4. *Best of Health & Fitness* (Beaverton, Ore.: Skies America Publishing Company and Cabe Communications, Inc., 1996), 15.

5. Margolis and Kostuik, *Low Back Pain*, 27.

CHAPTER 4

Your Spine at Work, At Home, and On the Telephone

1. Quoted in 1998 class notes by Marjorie Werrell, president of Ergoworks Consulting, Gaithersburg, Md.

2. These suggestions come from Carol Krucoff, "Putting Stress on Hold," *Washington Post*, August 26, 1997, Health Section.

3. "Ergolines," *Ergoworks Newsletter*, Gaithersburg, Md., Winter 1997.

CHAPTER 5

Oh, For a Good Night's Sleep

1. Gallup Poll, 1991.

2. *Wake Up America*, Report of the National Commission on Sleep Disorders Research (NCSDR), Executive Summary, Vol. 1, January, 1993, vi.

3. Reprinted by permission from *The Better Sleep Guide*, The Better Sleep Council, 1996, 3. Also available at <www.bettersleep.org>.

4. Rick Weiss, "Wake Up, Sleepy Teens," *Washington Post*, September 9, 1997, Health Section, 8.

5. Survey conducted by American Society of Chartered Life Underwriters & Chartered Financial Consultants and the Ethics Officer Association; quoted in *Washington Post*, September 14, 1997.

6. Orman, "Guide to Better Sleep," TRO Publications, 2936 E. Baltimore St., Baltimore, MD 21224; Web: <www.stresscure.com>.

7. Weiss, "Wake Up, Sleepy Teens," Health Section, 8.

8. American Academy of Otolaryngology—Head and Neck Surgery, Inc., Alexandria, VA 22314-3357; Web: <www.entnet.org>.

9. *Are You Getting the Sleep You Need?* (Carthage, Mo.: Leggett & Platt, Inc., 1995), 7.

10. Hilde Hartnett, "If Counting Sheep Fails...," AARP Bulletin, December 1996, 2.

11. *Wake Up America*, Report of NCSDR, 33.

12. *The Good Night Guide*, Better Sleep Council, 1993, 18.

13. Dr. Oexman is Director of Ergonomics Research for Leggett & Platt, P.O. Box 757, Carthage, MO 64836.

14. Quoted in material supplied by the Better Sleep Council.

15. *Wake Up America*, Report of NCSDR, vi.

16. Harris H. McIlwain, M.D., and Debra Fulghum Bruce, *The Fibromyalgia Handbook* (New York: Henry Holt and Co., 1996), 123.

17. Arlene Eisenberg, Heidi E. Murkoff, Sandee E. Hathaway, *What to Expect When You're Expecting* (New York: Workman Publishing Co., 1996), 173.

18. Ibid., 173.

CHAPTER 6
How to Buy a Mattress or a Whole New Bed

1. For additional material on determining whether you need a new mattress, check The Better Sleep Council's Web site: <www.bettersleep.org>.

2. "Sweet Dreams are Made of This," *New York Times*, October 2, 1997, C4.

3. Ibid.

4. "Sweet Dreams?" *Consumer Reports*, March 1997, 20.

5. "Sweet Dreams," *New York Times*, C4.

6. Clinical Physiology Research Dept., Lillhagen Hospital, Gothenburg, Sweden, 1993.

CHAPTER 7
The Many Forms of Arthritis

1. Simeon Margolis, M.D., Ph.D., and John A. Flynn, M.D., *The Johns Hopkins White Papers: Arthritis* (New York: Medletter Associates, Inc., 1997), 28.

2. Ibid., 6.

3. Jason Theodosakis, M.D., M.S., M.P.H.; Brenda Adderly, M.H.A.; and Barry Fox, Ph.D., *The Arthritis Cure* (New York: St. Martin's Griffin, 1998), 11.

4. McIlwain and Bruce, *The Fibromyalgia Handbook* (New York: Henry Holt and Co., Inc., 1996).

5. Theodosakis et al., loc. cit.

6. Drs. Christiane Northrup, Andrew Weil, and Simeon Margolis.

7. Norman Cousins, *Anatomy of an Illness* (New York: Bantam, 1979), 39.

8. Theodosakis et al., *The Arthritis Cure*, 83.

9. Margolis and Flynn, 61.

CHAPTER 8

Carpal Tunnel Syndrome and Repetitive Motion Injuries

1. BLS data are from 1994.

2. Sarah Glazer, "A Modern Malady," *Washington Post*, March 12, 1996, Health Section, 15.

3. Jacqueline L. Salmon, "For Students, Painful Lesson on Computers," *Washington Post*, May 17, 1998, 1.

4. Glazer, 15.

5. Alex Pirie and Hollis Herman, *How to Raise Children Without Breaking Your Back* (Somerville, Mass.: IBIS Publications, 1995), 133.

CHAPTER 9

Back Care in Daily Life

1. Eisenberg et al., *What to Expect When You're Expecting*, 174–5.

2. Alex Pirie and Hollis Herman (Somerville, Mass.: IBIS Publications, 1995).

3. Ibid., 23.

4. Available at JoAnne's Bed and Back Shops. Or contact Dr. Mort Orman, TRO Productions, Inc., 2936 E. Baltimore St., Baltimore, MD 21224, or his Web site: <www.stresscure.com>.

5. (Berkeley, Calif.: Rodmell Press, 1992).

6. Sold in JoAnne's Bed and Back Shops, or available from Jerome Cutting Corp., 601 West 26 St., New York, NY 10001.

I N D E X

Sleepwalking, 84, 88
Smith, Mark, 44
Snoring, 87, 88
Spinal stenosis, 47
Spine
    aging of, 41
    pain in, 40
    see also Back pain; Neck pain
Spondylolysis, 47
Sprains, 49
Strains, 49
Stress
    as cause of pain, 40, 50
    management, 145-146
    sleep and, 92
Stretch Break™, 135
Stretching, 30, 33, 57, 61-62
Stretching (book), 33, 61, 143
Swayback. See Lordosis
Swedish foam. *See* E-Foam™

Target heart rate, 31
Teeth gnashing. *See* Bruxism

Telephone posture tips, 77-78
Theodosakis, Jason, 119, 123
Thoracic curve, 48
Thoracic Outlet Syndrome, 133
TMJ, 43
Travel, tips for, 142-144
Tribole, Evelyn, 29

Vertebrae, 46, 48

Water beds, 103, 121
Weil, Andrew, 36
Werrell, Marjorie, 40, 71
What to Expect When You're Expecting, 138
Wrist health guidelines, 134-136

Yoga, 34, 57, 122, 146-147
Yo-yo dieting, 28